The
Empowered
Hysterectomy

The Empowered Hysterectomy

Your Complete Handbook
to Diagnosis, Decision,
and Treatment

Kameelah Phillips, MD

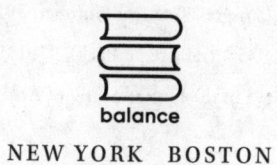

balance

NEW YORK BOSTON

The information herein is not intended to be a substitute for medical advice. You are advised to consult with your health care professional with regard to matters relating to your health, and in particular regarding matters that may require diagnosis or medical attention.

Balance
Hachette Book Group
1290 Avenue of the Americas
New York, NY 10104
GCP-Balance.com
@GCPBalance

First Edition: May 2025

Balance is an imprint of Grand Central Publishing. The Balance name and logo are registered trademarks of Hachette Book Group, Inc.

The publisher is not responsible for websites (or their content) that are not owned by the publisher.

Balance books may be purchased in bulk for business, educational, or promotional use. For information, please contact your local bookseller or the Hachette Book Group Special Markets Department at special.markets@hbgusa.com.

Print book interior design by Timothy Shaner, NightandDayDesign.biz

Illustrations by Carol Hrejsa, copyright © 2025 Balance

Library of Congress Control Number: 2025932838

ISBNs: 9781538769355 (trade paperback), 9781538769362 (ebook)

Printed in the United States of America

LSC-C

Printing 1, 2025

To my friends and family, whose love, support, and unwavering belief in me have carried me through every challenge.

To my patients, whose courage and resilience inspire me daily—you are the heart of this work.

To the millions of women around the world navigating the complexities of their bodies—this book is for you.

May it serve as an empowering guide as you make decisions rooted in knowledge, confidence, and self-love.

And to every person who has ever doubted their strength or silenced their voice—may this book remind you that you are powerful, deserving, and never alone.

With gratitude and hope,
KPC

A Note from the Author

Throughout this book I have tried to be intentional in my use of gendered language and inclusive of the needs of transgender and gender-fluid individuals, but this can get tricky when citing study results and discussing anatomy. I encourage the reader to think expansively when it comes to these descriptions and to consider their own specific needs and unique relationship to their bodies and their gender.

Contents

Part Three: If You Opt to Have a Hysterectomy

The
Empowered
Hysterectomy

Introduction

Taking Your Power Back

My friends and patients often ask me why I became an obstetrician-gynecologist and for a long time it was challenging to articulate. It never seemed like a choice, but more like a calling I followed from a young age. I was raised by strong, resilient women—my grandmother, Louise, my mother, Cynthia, and my devoted aunts. They were the foundation of my life. They dedicated their lives to not only supporting me, but also my entire family. These were the same women who also battled a host of reproductive health issues—fibroids, pelvic pain, and heavy bleeding—and when they suffered, my entire family felt it. I watched as my mother and aunts silently fought to hold everything together—our family, our lives, and themselves—while quietly managing their health struggles.

At an early age, I came to understand that when the women of the family are not well, the entire family suffers, and this has a ripple effect that touches the entire community. Over the years, these memories guided my path in medicine and eventually led me to become an ob-gyn. As an ob-gyn, I not only take care of women who were much like my grandmother, mother, and aunts—women who carry the weight of the family on their shoulders—I also take care of families and entire communities by helping women who would otherwise silently battle fibroids,

1

endometriosis, pelvic pain, and abnormal bleeding. I have seen the impact these conditions have on their lives—missed days at work, lost opportunities, relationships put on hold, and dreams delayed. I have lost track of how many times women have entered my office in tears after being told to "just have a hysterectomy," even if they were in the prime of their reproductive years, still hoping to have children, or simply wanting more options. It is heartbreaking to see how many women society and medicine have conditioned to believe that suffering is simply part of being a woman, that pain and heavy bleeding are just things we have to live with, and that relief comes only with silence, compliance, and even drastic measures.

I want you to know it doesn't have to be this way. We all know that historically, women's pain has been dismissed and minimized, labeled "hysterical," and "crazy," even made up. It often takes years, sometimes decades, to receive the right diagnosis and the right care. This book is my effort to do better for you—to align the best of our current treatment options with your personal health goals, whether that's preserving fertility, resolving heavy bleeding, living pain-free, or all of the above. I want to help you make choices you feel good about. I want you to feel empowered enough in your own knowledge that you're better able to trust your doctors and know that they have your best interest at heart. I want to equip you with the information you need to make educated and empowered decisions for yourself.

I know that medicine and doctors have a long way to go in earning your trust back.

Each year, approximately 600,000 women have a hysterectomy. By any account, this is a huge number. Now there are truly situations where a hysterectomy can be one of the best decisions of your life—when it is your choice, when it aligns with your needs, and when you are fully informed about your options. The truth is, though, that too many women, especially women of color, disabled women, low-income women, unsuspecting women, are steered toward hysterectomies without understanding all their options. Too often women, including my mother and aunts, are rushed into a decision that forever changes their bodies and their lives, without the information they deserve. To me this is heartbreaking.

This book is for those who hold everyone else's lives together, placing their own needs on the back burner while their own health suffers until they are convinced that a hysterectomy is the only answer. We have collectively been gaslit by medicine and society—both of whom tell us to either deal with it or "just take it out." Neither answer is acceptable without exploring the options and the nuance between these extremes.

Trans men and nonbinary folks seeking gender-affirming reproductive care also face a medical system that doesn't fully understand and appreciate the nuance of their lives. Similarly, the medical system fails to offer critical and pertinent information they deserve when making decisions about their bodies. This is also not acceptable.

You deserve to have a voice in your healthcare, to feel confident making the choices that are right for you, and to live a life free from unnecessary suffering. This is your life and your body. I am privileged to walk beside you as you explore your options every step of the way.

Welcome to *The Empowered Hysterectomy*. Let's take this journey together.

Love,

Dr. Kameelah Phillips

PART ONE

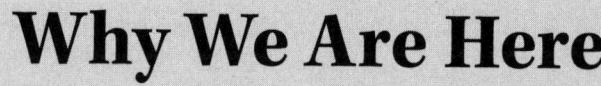

Why We Are Here

1

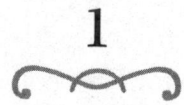

Misunderstood and Medicalized

The Uterus, a History of Stigma and Control

In the middle of the flanks of women lies the womb,
a female viscus, closely resembling an animal.
—Aretaceus of Cappadocia

I still remember my first connection with my uterus. I was twelve years old and on a grand adventure with my favorite uncle, Greg. Every summer, I would go with him for Family Day on the massive United States Navy carrier, the USS *Kitty Hawk*. When I took a break from the festivities to go to the bathroom, I discovered red stains in my underwear. I knew exactly what this was. Well, I thought, what perfect timing. My first period on a day surrounded by sailors, airplanes, and the wide-open Pacific Ocean. My mother had suggested that my period may start soon, but being in the middle of the Pacific Ocean on a "men's only" vessel was definitely not what I imaged. Thankfully she had given me the heads-up so I didn't panic. I found my uncle Greg, leaned in and whispered in his ear that I had started my period. I still remember the look of panic and pallor that swept over his face. He was out of his league but sprang into action. He rushed to find a Navy wife to help me. I never knew her name, but this "auntie" took me under her wing and guided me to the steel, bare-bones Navy latrine. Here she showed me how to fashion my first pad—straight from good ol' government-issued toilet paper.

After we docked, we hurried home. I could not wait to share the news with my mom and beloved aunts. Finally, I was a woman. Their first words in response to my news were, "Aww, I'm sorry." I was confused. Wait, what? I had waited my whole (okay, admittedly short) life for this moment. I finally got my period and they were apologizing? My mom and aunt could sense my disappointment in their lackluster response. And because they are phenomenal women, they made it up to me that weekend by throwing me a surprise Period Party—the same celebration of womanhood that I read about in all my preteen coming-of-age books. I was over the moon.

Within a few months, though, my relationship with my period grew complicated. Every month like clockwork, my uterus delivered my period—no, really, sometimes down to the very hour—and with my period came the three days of life-altering nausea, vomiting, and pain. I finally understood my aunt's apology. Three months into womanhood, I was sorry, too.

Does this story feel familiar? Was this you growing up? I hear a story like this every day in my gynecology practice and it never fails to amaze me how similar we all are when it comes to our menstrual cycle. For many of us, our relationships with our reproductive organs—specifically our uterus—start at a young age and evolves over time. And let's keep it real: for many seasons it can be a very love-hate relationship. If you're reading this book then chances are you don't feel very warm and fuzzy about your uterus right now. I hear you. You are just like most of my patients—both fascinated and frustrated by their bodies. On the one hand, you are eager to have a deeper understanding of your health yet, on the other hand, you are struggling with the idea that your body has betrayed you.

The road to understanding and managing issues of the uterus and your reproductive health is complex and emotional. This is not just a medical issue—it is deeply personal, cultural, and political too. Often it is impossible to tease apart the intersection of all these parts of yourself. But, before we dive into the physiological, biological, and medical details of your uterine health journey or decision to have a hysterectomy, let's take a pause to understand the uterus itself. Who is she? What is she capable of? What is the historical and cultural context that has us in turmoil and at odds with the medical establishment and our bodies? The uterus is a powerful organ and the center of your reproductive and sexual health. So, it makes sense that when something is going on with your body, it can have a huge effect on your quality of life and that the decision to remove this organ is a big one.

But what exactly is the uterus and why is it so important? To understand both the strength and struggle, we need to take a basic look at what the uterus does and doesn't do and how it connects with the rest of your body. Understanding the anatomy, physiology, and the real-life implications of having a uterus is crucial. It is with this foundation that we can unpack the complexity of this powerhouse organ in your pelvis and why it has such a hold on our health and well-being.

The Amazing but Complex Uterus

Uterus is the Latin word meaning "womb" and anatomically speaking is the organ tucked behind your bladder and in front of your rectum. Unlike other parts of the reproductive system that come in pairs—the ovaries, fallopian tubes, and teste—there is only *one* uterus. This distinction alone establishes the uterus as a special organ, a standout in the world of reproduction, responsible for the revered role of initiating, protecting, and supporting the development of human life. For all the legislation and commotion surrounding the uterus, you will be surprised to learn that it is a pretty small organ. If you clench your fist, you are roughly approximating the size of a normal, nonpregnant uterus. To use a gynecologist's favorite comparison tool—fruit—you can also think of the uterus as about the size and shape of a pear. This pear is capable of big things. During pregnancy, the uterus will undergo a huge transformation. By the time of delivery, the uterus will be approximately twenty times larger than its original size due to growth and stretching of the muscle fibers. So, our little pear grows, over the course of ten months, to the size of a watermelon, and then returns to its previous size within several weeks of giving birth. This is a magical transformation; no other organ in your body has this capability. The uterus's ability to expand, contract, expand, and contract over and over again makes the uterus such a fascinating (and frustrating) organ.

While the uterus is small, do not confuse its size for its strength. Its unique construction—an intricate layered weave of spiraling muscle fibers—allows the uterine muscles to squeeze, twist, spiral, and push with such an intense strength that it can propel a baby out into the world and bring a grown woman to her knees when on your period. According to the book of *Guinness World Records*, the jaw (masseter) muscle is the strongest muscle in the body, but Guinness has clearly not spoken with a menstruating person on the second day of their period or for that matter, anyone enduring an unmedicated birth. Let's just say, if you have experienced either, you may have a different take on the strongest muscle in the body. Move over masseter; there is a new queen in town.

Not only is the uterus physically powerful, historically she is revered across cultures for what she can create. Your uterus is the only organ that can grow another organ. The placenta is a rich, life-sustaining organ that has several functions: it supports and protects a pregnancy, exchanges nutrients between and connects the mother and a growing fetus. And, when its mission is complete, the uterus expertly expels the fully formed placenta from the body—again, no other organ can do this.

The word *placenta* is Latin for "cake," Greek for "flat, slablike" and German for "mother cake" —all referring to the placenta's classic appearance. Typically, after a delivery, I inspect the placenta. The family is so excited and curious to see what it looks like and how it works. I always hear *oohs* and *ahhs* when showing a family the placenta, with its radiating vessels like the roots of a hundred-year-old tree. Every placenta is unique. This reverence has been lost in Western medicine, which tends to dismiss the placenta as medical waste. Meanwhile, cultures all over the world honor this vascular tree as a symbol of life, strength, longevity, and fertility. In some African cultures the placenta is viewed as the second baby and is often given a formal burial, while some Chinese communities ceremoniously eat the placenta after birth or use dried placenta to treat coughs, male impotence, and liver disease. These rituals remind us that long before "Western medicine" the uterus and placenta held significant cultural reverence for generations around the world.

While many of us have come to detest our menstruation, there is a hidden superpower in your menstrual blood, too, and you and the uterus do not get nearly enough credit for it. Your monthly—or perhaps even more frequent—visitor is a powerful potential source of lifesaving stem cells. I know what you are thinking. Menstrual blood and saving lives were not on this year's bingo card, but likely because we have been conditioned to treat our menses as uncomfortable and awkward. But here is the thing—cutting-edge research is exploring menstrual blood as a new, noninvasive source of stem cells. As you know, when pregnancy does not occur, the endometrial lining sheds as your monthly period. This lining is not just tissue and blood, but powerful, stem-cell rich fluid. What does this mean for you and science? Underneath the inconvenience of bleeding and the curse of cramps, every woman of reproductive age is the source of a renewable, ethical source of stem cells that have the potential to treat conditions like diabetes, endometriosis, skin disease, and neurodegenerative conditions like Parkinson's disease.

Your uterus has superpowers in ways we are just beginning to imagine—even when it doesn't feel this way.

But if the culture is still not ready to give the uterus her due R-E-S-P-E-C-T, let's talk about sex and its role in sexual pleasure. Did that get your attention? As gynecologists we talk about sex all the time—at least we should. To be clear, it is crucially important for women who have sex to experience orgasm and pleasure from sex. For many women this sensation originates at the clitoris and travels outward like fireworks for a total body experience. For some, an orgasm is not limited to the clitoris but travels deeper into the cervix and uterus. Researchers have found that during sex, there is an increase in blood flow to the uterus and the pelvis. This helps the uterus to actively rise up and out of the lower pelvis to make way for vaginal penetration. Remarkably, for some women, the unmistakable waves of orgasmic pleasure come from contractions originating in the uterus and cervix. Your uterus is not passive in your sexual experience and the connection between the uterus, pleasure, and sex is something to keep in mind as we talk more about hysterectomy. More than just an organ to nurture and grow babies or cause monthly distress, your uterus can be a source of sexual pleasure, connection, and empowerment.

Celebrating the Uterus—with Cake

Every year when we gather to celebrate a birthday, let us remember that we are also honoring the placenta—the original "cake" that nourished us in the womb and marked the beginning of our earth side journey.

You're Not Crazy, It's Just Your Uterus (According to the Ancient Origins of Medicine)

In my practice, I'm constantly in awe of how powerful the uterus is and at the same time deeply saddened by the havoc she can wreak in my patients' lives. What complicates this journey even more is that nothing in women's health is ever straightforward. More than just a body part, the uterus is also a symbol, entangled in politics, social commentary, economic trends, technology, cultural shifts, and even medical beliefs that have evolved (or not evolved) over time. From puberty through our fertile years, and even in menopause, the symbolism of the uterus is profound. So while I can tell you that your uterus creates and protects life, is a vital source of pleasure, and is the most unique organ in the human body, it may be hard to accept when we are in pain and troubled by her existence.

Long before modern medicine, ancient cultures as far back as Egypt understood the social and cultural power of the womb. It was a source of life, healing, and a connection to deeper mystical forces. However, over time, it also came to be viewed as something to control, manage, and even fear. So, when you are trying to figure out what is going on with your body, how to manage your symptoms, or even whether or not to have a hysterectomy, subconsciously none of this process or decision-making is happening in a vacuum.

We know the uterus hasn't always been treated with the deference she deserves. The very origins of medicine, including gynecology, emerged not only from the idea that the uterus was pathologic, but also from the need to commodify both the female body and the reproductive organs. How we have come to understand our bodies, the uterus, and our reproductive health is deeply rooted in a history of patriarchy, capitalism, and the evolving tradition of medicine.

If we take a trip back to the earliest recorded times, we can see evidence that the uterus was not only just misunderstood but actually blamed for major illness. Philosophers like Aristotle, Soranus, Hippocrates (yes, the author of the Hippocratic Oath that all doctors take to do no harm) and others from this crew formed medicine's early beliefs about the fields of mental health and neurology, or the study of disorders of the nervous system. Surprise, surprise: they claimed that every problem in the female human body could somehow be traced back to the fault of your uterus. Feeling depressed? Blame the uterus. Feeling anxious? Blame the uterus. Having seizures? Blame the uterus.

For these "fathers" of medicine, the uterus was a bad actor. In early medical texts, the "wandering womb" theory suggested that the uterus caused illness by traveling throughout the body and wreaking havoc on other organs. Early medical texts used the Greek term for "wild beast" to refer to the uterus, perpetuating the commonly held notion of the female body as untamed and animalistic—a ticking time bomb in need of control. They believed that as the uterus grew in pregnancy it caused "hysterical suffocation," a concept that the uterus smothered organs in the body making it difficult to swallow, breathe, and causing stomach issues. Of course, a full-term uterus can cause difficulty breathing, swallowing, and digesting food by pressing up against your internal organs; we know now this is normal physiology and today would be described as normal third trimester pregnancy symptoms to me, but hey, what do I know?

Hysterical suffocation was also associated with seizures (probably eclampsia, a condition in pregnant women that causes high blood pressure and seizures), heart problems, and the onset of mental ailments like anxiety and depression (both unfortunately also common in pregnant women). So, while yes, your uterus may in fact drive you crazy, mental illness is not exclusive to the female body nor is it caused by your reproductive organs. Yet because these "Fathers of Medicine" used medical language to blame the uterus for mental illness and other ailments, this meant that only women could suffer from these "hysterical" events. The perceived power of the uterus was so strong that any distress or illness was labeled "hysterical" from the Greek word *hystera*, which means "uterus." This is where the term *hysteria* comes from—the idea that the uterus made women crazy.

Unfortunately, these negative and misguided theories persisted, and actually became more sophisticated and widespread. From ancient times through the medieval period and into the European Renaissance these concepts became the foundation of the fields of psychiatry, medicine, medical education, and popular culture branding women as "hysterical," unstable, and biologically inferior versions of men. These theories set the foundation for the gaslighting women experience in the medical space. Have you ever been told "you're not having pain, it's all in your head" or "it's just stress" or "you just need to lose weight?" This attitude directly descends from the early linking of the uterus to female mental health. In the early 2000s, even some of my male medical school professors would gaslight female patients by suggesting that their experience and endometriosis itself wasn't real; it was just a group of women overreacting or being dramatic about their period cramps. Imagine that—thousands of years after the "wandering womb" and "hysterical suffocation," I—an impressionable medical student—was still being taught that women should be told that their very real pain was just a figment of their imagination.

But wait—there is so much more to this story. The migration of people from Europe to the Americas represented a turning point in the field of medicine. From the 1600s onward, the field of medicine became heavily embedded in the role of American chattel slavery. Medicine—an institution already deeply entrenched in sexism and patriarchy—now became layered with institutionalized racism. It is under this multilayered web of oppression that the American medical establishment developed into what we know today. More specifically, it is during this time that the field of modern obstetrics and gynecology flourished—yes, unequivocally on the pain and suffering of Black enslaved women who birthed this field.

The Birth of Obstetrics and Gynecology

Growing up, whenever my aunts or mother were struggling with heavy bleeding from fibroids, or my grandmother wasn't feeling well, the responsibility of my care went to my maternal grandfather, Jimmy, or Papa as I called him. Now while I loved him dearly, and he did his best, Papa wasn't much for hair braiding so I would often go to school with my hair a total mess, and dinner was less appealing than what I was accustomed to. Despite this, while he would attempt to do my hair he would tell me stories, because at his core, my papa was an educator and scholar. He was an expert on American history, particularly American chattel slavery, and together we would sit for hours in his library reading books. It was with him that I learned about the painful origins of the field I hoped to study.

As early as 1526, the transatlantic slave trade forcibly brought African men, women, and children to the Americas. Lasting hundreds of years, it was the largest forced migration of human beings—bringing ten to thirteen million people to provide human labor to build the United States. With time, the moral climate around enslavement changed and by 1808, the official end of the transatlantic slave trade was declared. While on paper the trading of enslaved people ended—we know that enslavement in the American colonies quietly and illegally continued. With the flow of new human capital interrupted and a nation dependent on enslaved labor to support the cotton, tobacco, textile, sugar, rice, cocoa, coffee, and a host of other industries, owners of enslaved people searched for ways to sustain their workforce. This is when the economic value of enslaved women became exceedingly clear. To sustain the workforce, enslaved women were not simply laborers, they were the only source of ongoing human capital. These women were both workers and birthers of the next enslaved generation. This shift meant owners had an economic incentive to optimize enslaved women's fertility and their ability to birth healthy babies. It is in this context that women's health, maternal healthcare, and the field of obstetrics—the medical science that deals with pregnancy, birth, and the postpartum period—was born.

Until this time, the work of birthing was traditionally gender-based. In almost every culture all things fertility, pregnancy, or birth was considered women's work; in fact it was considered taboo for a man to be present during labor or birth. Birth workers were midwives, priestesses, and local healers whose knowledge was passed down from generation to generation. This tradition was no different in colonial America where midwifery was a highly regarded practice. Experienced midwives that survived the Middle Passage to the Americas used their ancestral knowledge about reproductive health and birth from their native lands in their local communities. However, as the pressure to grow the enslaved workforce grew, the role of midwifery and "women's work" changed. Enslavers became increasingly aware that midwives and enslaved women used practices to control their fertility and even induce abortion. Ancestral practices that were once held in esteem by enslavers were now viewed as suspicious, backward, and a threat to the growth of their enslaved workforce.

The role of midwives and their craft soon came under attack, fueled by the rise of young, newly educated, white male physicians who were eager to curry favor with plantation owners by offering solutions to support the growth of the enslaved population. These young physicians actively delegitimized midwifery, labeling their practices as dirty and unsophisticated. They attributed the high infant and maternal death rate to midwives' "unsanitary and superstitious" practices—and, ahem, not the brutality of slavery. During a time of little oversight and regulation, these new physicians were desperate to do hands-on medical work in order to further their understanding of anatomy and physiology. For them, "women's issues" proved to be a lucrative area for medical exploration and financial gain. Fertility, pregnancy, and the female body—once an area dominated by women—suddenly became the new frontier for medical and surgical experimentation.

As you can imagine, enslaved women faced difficult pregnancies. Often pregnant during their teenage years, their young bodies were undernourished and harshly treated. Pregnancy for an enslaved women was a dangerous venture. Long, obstructed labor, poor nutrition, and abysmal living conditions often resulted in severe injuries or death to the enslaved woman and her baby. One particularly horrific yet common labor-related complication of labor that enslaved women experienced is a vesicovaginal fistula (VVF). This occurs when the baby's head remains pressed on the cervix, bladder, and vagina for an extended amount of time. The constant and prolonged compression of the head on the bladder and vagina reduces blood flow to the area and can cause the tissue to die and create a tunnel from the bladder to the vagina. This connection leads to a constant, uncontrollable leakage of urine from the vagina. While a VVF is not fatal, it is life changing in the worst way. Imagine the horror of constant smell and pain these women suffered not to mention the loss of human dignity. To the enslaver, VVF rendered the enslaved woman "useless" for household chores, unable to work in fields, or bear more children. Her "property" value as an enslaved person was irreparably diminished.

It is in this setting that the growing body of inexperienced white male doctors exploited the bodies of enslaved women to birth the field of gynecology—the medical specialty that deals with the health of the female reproductive system, including the breasts, genitals, and pelvic organs. Enter the most famous among these—Dr. J. Marion Sims, also known as the "father of gynecology."

As an aspiring doctor, Dr. Sims built his home and hospital conveniently near a large enslaved person's trading post in Montgomery, Alabama. Over a five-year span he recorded his revolving door of experimental procedures on enslaved women with VVF. His records note countless enslaved women who moved in and out of this hospital. Three teenagers in particular, Anarcha (aged seventeen), Lucy (aged seventeen), and Betsey (aged eighteen)—suffered upward of thirty surgeries at the hands of Dr. Sims. His journals documented their extreme pain while the enslaved women restrain one another during his procedures all of which were performed without anesthesia—although it was available during this time. After perfecting his technique, Dr. Sims went on to perform this procedure on white women across the American Northeast and Europe, this time with anesthesia.

The Civil War ended in 1865 and with it the institution of slavery. The institutionalized system of exploitation of African American women didn't stop, however, it just changed its face. When the US could no longer benefit from enslaved labor, the country shifted its focus toward controlling fertility and limiting the population of formerly enslaved people in the United States. This legacy of abuse started under the guise of medical care, and ranged from forced sterilizations of poor, Black, brown, and Indigenous women to the infamous "Mississippi appendectomy," a common practice in the Southern states wherein Black women would enter the hospital for one procedure—maybe the removal of their appendix—and be given a hysterectomy without their knowledge or consent. The 1950s, sixties, and seventies brought the eugenics movement and contraception studies to poor communities of color, where participants were unaware of the potential complications or side effects of the hormonal contraception they were taking. Can you begin to understand why so many women, especially Black, brown, and Indigenous women, are skeptical and outright distrustful of the medical community?

Talking about the history of gynecology and medicine makes me angry and heartbroken. You may be thinking, "Does this really matter? I picked up this book because I need help with my hysterectomy." Here is the thing: nothing happens in isolation. Have you ever walked into your gynecologist's office with a pit in your stomach and wonder why? Have you ever wondered why it is only recently that there's been an outcry for proper pain management during gynecological procedures like IUD insertions? Or why Black women are three to four times more likely to die from pregnancy-related complications than white women—in some areas this figure climbs to twelve times more? Why do women, especially Black women, receive less pain management in the ER or face higher rates of hysterectomies in this country? The roots of these disparities trace back to a deeply flawed and racist healthcare system—one that deemed it acceptable to operate on enslaved Black women without anes-thesia. It stems from the notion that women's pain is in their head or caused by their reproductive organs. These beliefs have created a narrative that has shaped gynecology and women's health. These systemic injustices persist, echoing through time and shape the inequities we still confront today.

These origins ingrained harmful beliefs within the medical community: that women—especially minority women—can endure unspeakable pain; that women's bodies are fair grounds for experimentation; and that male doctors inherently know more or better about your body than you do. Think about it—would we ever expect men to undergo any genital procedure without pain relief? No, of course not.

Today, the echoes of this history still shape our present. It shows up in the fragmented patriarchal doctor-patient relationship that makes many of us dread going to the doctor's office. They are present in the billions of dollars poured into medical research, with only a sliver dedicated to women's health. They are felt in the lives of endometriosis patients who are told, "It's all in your head" and who see an average of eight physicians before their condition is properly diagnosed. The ripple effect of this origin story is far reaching and deeply embedded in our culture, touching the lives of all women in ways both seen and unseen.

A Different Way Forward

Gynecology was born in an era when women were stripped of their autonomy—when decisions about our own bodies were made for us, not by us. The expectation was, and still often is, that you simply follow doctor's orders. Your experience is heavily rooted in patriarchal beliefs about women's bodies as well as the economic value of controlling them. Let me be clear-this is not in your head. You are right. You are not always given all the options. It's not new, but my goal, my mission, is to make sure it ends here. If you've picked up this book it's likely that you or someone you love has experienced years if not decades of bleeding, pain, and unanswered questions. You deserve more than just a simple "yes" or "no" or someone telling you what to do when it comes to the very serious decision about whether or not to have a hysterectomy. You deserve to make informed decisions about your body and your health. You deserve real conversations about every decision, no matter how small, every step of the way.

Medicine is broken. We all know it. You feel rushed during appointments with your questions often left unanswered and with an uncomfortable sense that your voice is not being heard. The truth is that most doctors entered medicine with the best of intentions—to educate, empower, and be partners in your health journey so that you can live your fullest and healthiest life. We want to learn about your health, deep dive into your concerns, and help guide you through these critical decisions—but we just can't do this in a fifteen-minute window.

In these pages, I'm going to take the time to teach you about your body, your symptoms, and the options available to treat your condition(s). Beyond that, I want to help you feel empowered to clearly articulate your values, needs, and concerns about your health. Let's face it—too often, physicians talk *at* us and not *to* us. I don't know about you, but this leaves me feeling upset, uncomfortable, and anxious. We are going to break down the confusing and frustrating medical jargon so you can confidently take the wheel as you navigate your way to better health.

Let's pause for a moment. We are not in your doctor's office right now. It's just me and you. Take a deep breath in and let it out. Unless you've been told you have a life-threatening condition and need swift action, you have time to learn, think, and plan. In fact, you've likely been dealing with these issues for years so taking the time to absorb what in this book will not delay or change your outcome—it will only improve the confidence in your decision-making. As a rule, I do not let patients schedule any surgery with me on our first meeting especially when we start discussing hysterectomy. This is your body, and no one should have to force or coerce you into surgery; *you* will know if and when you are ready. Don't let anyone rush you. Again, unless you have a medical emergency, give yourself permission to take the time you need to make this decision.

The key message I can leave you with is this: you are about to take your power back. This is not just for you, but for future generations and certainly for the ancestors who had no choice and were not given any options regarding their health. No more bleeding, pain, and suffering. No more medical gaslighting, coercion, or intimidation. Your voice is powerful. Your uterus is powerful. *You* are powerful.

It is time to reclaim your body, health, and future. Let's get going.

2

Know Thy Body

D on't tell anyone this story because it is kind of embarrassing, but about three years into my relationship with my husband, he walked into the bathroom just as I was about to flush the toilet. He glanced down, saw the deep maroon water swirling around the toilet bowl, and—with genuine concern—looked at me and said, "I don't understand how you all pee blood like that every month." Pause. I gave him *the look*. You know the side-eye and pursed lips combo more commonly known as "Black Girl's Face #103": *What in the entire world did this fool just say?* So many thoughts raced through my head, but I decided to be nice and settled on this: "Do you think I pee out of my vagina?" I asked, eyebrow raised. He quickly backpedaled with a nervous "No, no, no," and hurried out of the bathroom. And there it was: I realized my husband had absolutely no clue about basic female anatomy.

It got me wondering, do most of us—male or female—really know basic female anatomy? I grew up during a time when comprehensive and unbiased reproductive health information was a regular part of the school curriculum. As a young ob-gyn I often took for granted that anatomy was common knowledge. But now, after fifteen years of practicing medicine, I know better. Most of us, not just my husband, are riding the reproductive health struggle bus.

If I had a quarter for every time I hear, "Wait, my uterus does what?" or "The baby is coming out of where?" Well, you can imagine where my bank account would be by now. Women in their forties, fifties, and sixties—and the younger ones too—are woefully unfamiliar with their bodies. We don't know the correct terms for our body parts and are essentially disconnected from the reproductive health information that influences their lives and sexual health decisions.

So, this is what we must tackle first—the basics of your reproductive anatomy. It is crucial that you understand how your body works before someone offers to remove, alter, or leave something behind, right? Right. For far too long many of us have been bullied or shamed into ignorance about our bodies. This judgment-free refresher—or maybe first-time—mini anatomy course is going to help you reclaim the knowledge you may have lost or never had in the first place.

The Power of Words

Before we dive in, let's take a moment to talk about the power of words. You're going to learn a lot of medical terms for your body in the following pages and there's a reason for that. Many of us were raised calling our genitals vague, generic names like *private parts*, or learned cutesy euphemisms such as *hoo-ha, pee hole, fanny, vajayjay, lady parts, flower*. Trust me the list goes on and on. Research shows us that teaching our children and personally using appropriate medical terms for our respective body parts is a powerful tool. It builds body confidence and equips children with the language to report inappropriate behavior, which can help prevent sexual abuse.

Using the correct anatomical terms for all body parts, especially the genitals, not only fosters a healthy body image and self-esteem, it teaches us that our entire body is natural, normal, and worthy of respect. For adults, correct anatomical language is key to effectively communicate with everyone from your healthcare providers, partners, and even your own kids. Calling your body parts by their proper names isn't just about accuracy, it's about ownership. By owning the language of your body, you take the first step toward owning your health and your choices.

The Outer Structures: The Parts You Can See and Touch

In my office we have hand mirrors mounted on the wall in every room. We use them so patients can take a good look at their vulva and labia. I know it's awkward, and perhaps it's a little hard to read and look at the same time, but if you are in a private space go grab a mirror or use the camera on your phone so you can look at and touch these outer structures as we go through them—just don't forget to delete or hide any pictures you might snap. This is your chance to really see and connect with these parts of your body.

Start at the top of your vulva and move one section at a time, pausing to look, touch, and explore for as long as you would like. If this is your first time doing something like this feel free to giggle—I can understand how this may be a little uncomfortable. If it feels that way to you,

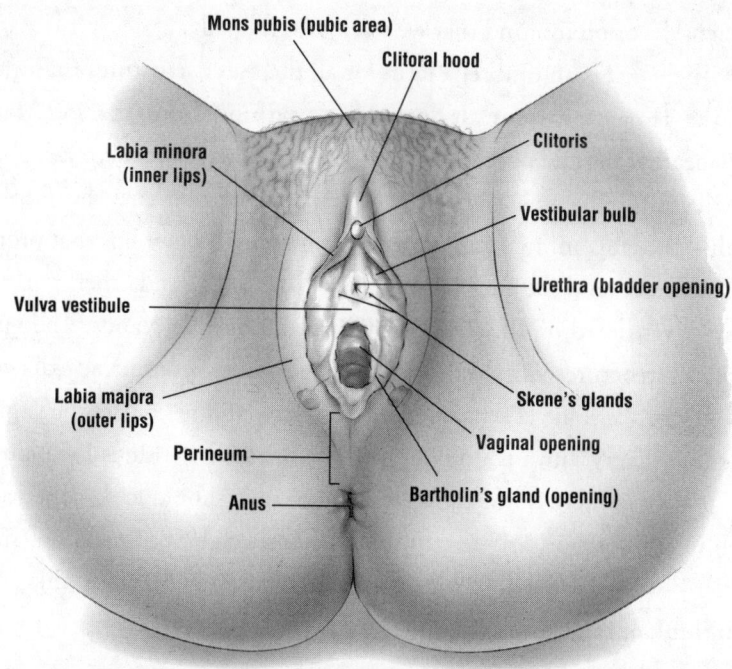

too, you are not alone. So go ahead: look, laugh, and even touch. It is your body—your personal playground—and getting to know it is both important and empowering.

The Vulva

Many of us use the words *vulva* and *vagina* interchangeably, but they are not the same. They are two unique and distinct structures so let's be specific. In over fifteen years of practice, I have come to firmly believe that understanding the vulva plays a crucial role in understanding and communicating about your body, sexuality, and even health conditions that may contribute to the reason you need this book.

Humans have been fascinated by the vulva since prehistoric times. Prehistoric engravings of the vulva in stone, ivory, and even mammoth molars show representations of the vulva far more frequently than images of the penis. Why? It's believed that while early civilizations may have had limited understanding of fertility—especially the male role—they recognized the undeniable power of the female body. It is with this ancient devotion in mind that we start with the vulva.

The *vulva* is an umbrella term for all the outer structures that make up the female anatomy. It includes everything from the soft, fatty, hair-bearing mound of tissue called the mons down to the skin just above the rectum. The vulva encompasses structures you may be familiar with—the labia minora and majora (the inner and outer lips that protect and comfort) and the clitoris and vaginal opening—and others you may have never heard of, like the Bartholin's and Skene's glands. The vulva protects structures like the urethra (the tube where your urine exits your body), the vestibule (a sensitive area of tissue), and of course, the vaginal opening. Every vulva is unique. It is one of the first things I explain to my patients. There is no "right" way your vulva should look—the variation in color, shape, and length makes you special. She is also not static either—your vulva will change with age. No two vulvas look alike. You can think of them as fingerprints—truly your personal calling card.

Mons Pubis

Now let's work from the top down, starting with the mons pubis. The mons is a fatty pad of triangle-shaped tissue located between the legs and right over the pubic bone. In my humble opinion, the mons receives the most scrutiny and judgment of all the vulvar parts for one primary reason: hair. As babies, we are born hairless, but after puberty this area becomes covered with thick, coarse hair. From an evolutionary perspective, pubic hair is a good thing! Hair helps protect our skin from infection, cushions the impact of penetration, and while invisible to the naked eye, small oil glands on the mons secrete pheromones to excite our partner during intimacy.

Yet, despite the marvels of evolution and because humans are humans, pubic hair has become political, so every decade or so the "socially acceptable" appearance of the mons gets a serious makeover. In the sixties and seventies, we appreciated a fuller, "bushy" look. The pubic hair was unrestricted and grew with wild abandon—likely how nature intended. In the eighties and nineties, pubic hair again became controversial, as magazines like *Playboy* and *Hustler* created a world forum for the scrutiny of the female body and the "landing strip," or the practice of removing all the hair from the front and the sides and leaving just a thin strip of pubic hair down the middle of the mons, became popular. More recently, the ubiquitous Brazilian wax leaves the mons totally bare. Whether you choose to trim, wax, or embrace your hair as it is, more power to you. Just know that pubic hair does serve a purpose so there is no shame in just letting it be.

Labia Majora and Minora

Just below the mons you will find the structures I like to consider a pair of sisters—not twins—called the labia majora and minora. Like the mons, these structures are also as unique as fingerprints. The labia majora, which literally means "large lips," are the outer skin folds of the vulva. Over the years, I have heard patients call the labia majora *fanny flaps*, *meat curtains*, and even *lady lips*—people can be so creative. Your labia majora start from the bottom of the mons pubis and travel along both sides of your vulva to the anus. Their primary job is to cover other sensitive vulvar structures and protect the labia minora—or small lips—which range from beautiful shades of light pink and mocha brown. Like the mons, the outer labia will become covered with coarse hair during puberty and special glands give each of us our unique scent. The labia majora are typically thick, wavy, and beautifully melanated. When the labia majora are gently parted, they reveal the labia minora, which tend to be long and thin. During sexual activity, the labia majora swell and become engorged with blood, which helps to cushion the pressure of penetration, making intimacy more comfortable.

Clitoris

Okay, if you've got your mirror or phone handy, sit with your legs slightly spread and gently open up your labia majora and minor to expose your clitoris. She is the queen of the vulva and sits proudly on top of her throne. Your clitoris has one job—pleasure. With over ten thousand nerve fibers there is no other structure in the body—male or female—whose sole purpose is sending shock waves through your body. Yes, it belongs all to you. *Well damn*, you say. Yes, it's true.

The visible part of the clitoris varies from person to person, ranging anywhere from the size of a pea to about the size of a thumb. But here is a surprise. This is just the tip of the iceberg. The clitoris actually extends under your skin on both sides of your vulva and—a little-known fun fact is that it measures up to five inches long on both sides. The size and abundance of nerve endings are what can make orgasm—for people who experience them—such an intense and mind-blowing experience. Nature gave her a hood, formed from the labia minora, to prevent constant stimulation when you walk or wipe. For those of you who like a little extra flair, this hood is what may be decorated with piercings—a patient of mine describes her clitoral hood ring as "a little bling" for her queen. You should definitely spend a moment to celebrate and get to know your clitoris. She is an incredible masterpiece of human anatomy—designed purely for your pleasure.

Urethra

The urethra is often confused with the vagina—not just by my husband. You would be surprised to know that many people (both male and female) do not know that the female genitals have three openings. No judgment, you are in good company, but let's set the record straight.

Your urethra is the first of the three openings moving downward from your mons. Located just south of the clitoris is the tube that allows urine to flow from your bladder and out of your body. It is hidden from sight unless the labia are opened—safely tucked away for protection. The urethra is not involved when you're considering a hysterectomy, but it's an important structure. Because its opening is small and very close proximity to the vagina, blood coming from the urethra can be mistaken for menstrual blood. If bleeding from the urethra is not properly diagnosed it can delay treatment for bladder conditions like kidney stones, urinary tract infections, and even bladder cancer. Just another reason why knowing your anatomy is so important for your health.

Vagina

A main player of the vulva, the vagina is the second opening on the mons. A quick brainstorm session can yield at least twenty euphemisms for this popular structure. Some are lovely and flattering and others downright disrespectful. On the one hand, she has little need for introduction, and on the other hand—as someone who sees vaginas every day—I'd argue she's underrated and misunderstood.

The vagina is an elastic, tubular, muscular structure that connects the vulva to the inner reproductive structures—the uterus and cervix. The opening of the vaginal canal is occasionally covered by a thin membrane called the hymen. The vagina has many functions. It is the passageway for menstrual blood that flows from the uterus and into the vagina. During penetrative intercourse with a male partner, the vagina is a reservoir for semen. Starting at the top of the vagina, semen then moves into the cervix, through the uterus, and eventually into the fallopian tubes.

Let's not forget that babies come out through the vagina, which can expand to accommodate childbirth and then return to her normal size. Additionally, the vagina provides access for surgical procedures like hysterectomy and a hysteroscopy—a simple procedure we will discuss later.

Aside from the structural and reproductive duties, the vagina is a great communicator. Vaginal discharge, odor, and bleeding are all communications about your health and what's going on inside. Her signals can tell you when something is "off" and it's time to visit the gynecologist.

Now that I've gotten all the official medical functions out of the way, permit me to be a little poetic. As someone who sees more vaginas than the average person, let me tell you she is perhaps your most unique and beautiful body part. Your vagina is dynamic, alive, and full of motion. Her walls are akin to the waves of the ocean. Like a Georgia O'Keeffe painting, the vagina is a mysterious and timeless beauty. A testament to both strength and beauty. She is not just a physical feature, but a symbol of strength, power, and resilience.

Perineum

While the perineum is not technically associated with the vulva, she is important and deserves a mention. You are probably familiar with the perineum, even if you didn't know it had a name. The perineum is the two-to-three-inch area of skin between the vaginal opening and the anal opening where the rectum starts. Its function is to connect the muscles of your vulva. The perineum is crucial. It can be injured during vaginal delivery and its integrity can impact urination and defecation if not properly repaired.

Rectum

While not an official structure of the vulva, we include the rectum because it's the third and final opening in your "down there" region. The rectum holds our stool until we are ready to use the bathroom. If you've ever had rectal fissures or hemorrhoids, you've experienced a literal pain in the butt. Bleeding can occur from the rectum, from internal and external hemorrhoids, fissures, and cancers. The rectum is also home to a lot of nerves, which make for sensitivity and pleasure.

Honorable Mention: Vulvar Vestibule

The vulvar vestibule is a special and distinct area on the vulva, not to be mistaken with the entire vulva. This region, which includes the urethral and vaginal openings and the surrounding skin, is marked by a noticeable change in appearance called Hart's line. In the vestibule area, there are two small openings on either side where a small set of glands (the Skene's glands) release moisture to protect the urethra and keep the vaginal area well lubricated.

* * *

If you're savvy, much of this may have been familiar to you, which is fabulous. Remember, this is about more than just anatomy—it's about empowerment. It's about owning your body. Your body is a source of strength, pleasure, and life, and the more you know her, the more confidently you can advocate for her. Let's keep going—there is so much more to explore.

Internal Structures—A Deep Dive into All the Stuff You Can't See

Having explored the external structures, it's time to go deeper into the mysterious and intricate reproductive anatomy nestled in the seat of your pelvis, often the root cause of "Why am I dealing with these [insert symptoms]?" This section will help you make sense of what's happening inside your body, so you can walk into your doctor's office confident, informed, and ready to advocate for yourself.

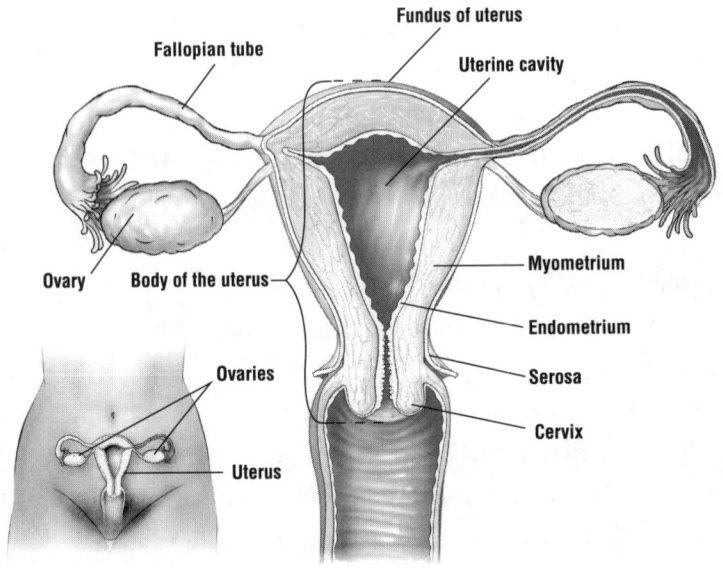

Cervix

If you have ever felt a "bump" deep in your—or someone else's—vagina, or felt like your partner is hitting something deep in your body during sex, you are most likely feeling your cervix. The cervix is where the upper part of the vagina and the lower part of the uterus meet and is important to your basic health. Your cervix is the star of the show during your annual Pap smear—the test that screens you for cervical cancer. She is the passageway for menstrual blood and cervical mucus—which you know if you have ever practiced fertility tracking can indicate ovulation—as well as semen. The cervix is typically firm, but during ovulation it will soften to allow sperm to enter the uterus.

Most of the time, the cervix remains closed and acts as a barrier to keep bacteria out of your uterus and the upper reproductive tract. During labor the cervix can open to ten centimeters wide—about the size of a cantaloupe—allowing babies to be born.

Interestingly, when you're sexually aroused your cervix and uterus move upward to elongate the vaginal canal during sex to accommodate penetration. Some people also receive pleasure when their cervix is stimulated or touched, making sexual pleasure an important consideration when discussing any surgery that can potentially impact the cervix.

Uterus

Your uterus, like your clitoris, is also a star of the reproductive health show—literally and figuratively the center of your reproductive system. It is both the center of your anatomy and a powerhouse of function. Sitting just above your cervix and vagina, it is flanked by your fallopian tubes and ovaries on either side.

As we discussed earlier, the uterus is uniquely powerful. Though it usually weighs about sixty grams (about the weight of a small kiwifruit), it can grow significantly during pregnancy or with conditions like fibroids, reaching the size of a watermelon. You can think of the uterus as a papaya—yes, a papaya. Stay with me here:

- The *serosa* (outer layer) is like the papaya's skin—it is smooth, thin, and covers the underlying muscle.
- The *myometrium* (muscular middle layer) is the fleshy part of the fruit where period cramps and labor contractions occur. It is a thicker muscular layer.
- The *endometrium* (inner lining) is the seeded cavity of the papaya. This is the uterine cavity where menstrual blood originates, babies grow, and where intrauterine devices (IUDs) are placed to prevent pregnancy.

Understanding these layers is crucial, especially when it comes to diagnosing symptoms and exploring treatment options. The layer where you have an issue—whether it's fibroids, polyps, or adenomyosis—will determine how you experience symptoms and how we treat them. So while the uterus may feel like "one big organ" the details matter when addressing your health.

What Are Polyps?

Polyps are abnormal tissue growths that can be found in many parts of the body. In the uterus or cervix, they are often small, long tubular or flat mushroom-shaped growths. While typically benign—not related to cancer—they can cause symptoms like heavy or irregular bleeding when on the cervix or inside the uterus. Polyps are typically removed to rule out cancer and resolve any symptoms they may cause such as heavy or irregular bleeding.

Fallopian Tubes

Fallopian tubes don't get much attention unless we're talking about pregnancy or even ovarian cancer. These spaghettilike tubes connect the uterus to the ovaries and are where the egg and sperm meet. The fimbriae are fingerlike projections at ends of the tube that collect the released egg and guide it into the fallopian tube to meet any waiting sperm. If the egg and sperm successfully meet and fertilize, they will continue to travel down the tube to eventually implant in the uterine cavity.

Occasionally a fertilized egg does not make it to the uterus and instead gets struck in the fallopian tube. This is an ectopic pregnancy and is a serious medical condition requiring immediate medical attention. Sometimes medicine can be used to treat an ectopic pregnancy, but in more advanced cases surgery may be required to remove either part of or the entire fallopian tube.

Removing the entire fallopian tube (a salpingectomy) is the most common surgical treatment for ectopic pregnancies. A common form of permanent contraception is the complete removal of the fallopian tube, commonly called a tubal ligation or "getting your tubes tied." While patients often use this phrase, your doctor does not really "tie" the tubes, so they can never be "untied." Current research also shows that many ovarian cancers may originate in the fimbriae. Because of this, the current standard of care is to remove the entire fallopian tube both for birth control purposes and during a hysterectomy to reduce your risk of ovarian cancer by up to 80 percent. This is now the standard for women at average risk of ovarian cancer and supported by several women's health organizations. If you opt for surgery, keeping or removing the fallopian tubes will be one of the important conversations you will have with your gynecologist before you proceed.

Ovaries

Finally, we reach the ovaries. There are two almond-shaped structures are slightly smaller than a golf ball and are essential to your reproductive health. The fact that there are two signals their importance. The ovaries have two major roles: they are responsible for storing your eggs and producing hormones such as estrogen, progesterone, and testosterone.

We are born with one to two million eggs, but by the time we reach puberty this number has dramatically decreased to about five hundred thousand. With each menstrual cycle, only one or two (as is the case for fraternal twins) eggs are ovulated. To get to this egg, however, about a thousand immature eggs are lost and reabsorbed during your monthly cycle. By age thirty-five, the rate of loss increases significantly.

Your ovaries start to awaken around puberty to produce the female hormones and then ramp down this production during perimenopause, eventually stopping after menopause. If your ovaries are removed before age forty, you will enter premature menopause (or a more abrupt menopause if you are already in perimenopause). This is important because the instantaneous drop in estrogen production influences your bone health and risk of heart disease. Understanding the importance of your ovaries and their role in estrogen, progesterone, and testosterone hormone production require careful consideration of your age, health, and future plans for hormone replacement.

Knowledge Is Power

If you are here, chances are you have had a challenging relationship with one or more of these body parts. Maybe you are considering surgery, and you're scared, confused, or feeling sad about removing any of them. Before we move on to the nitty-gritty about treatment options, I invite you to take a moment to celebrate how amazing the female body—including yours—truly is. I spend a lot of time with female reproductive anatomy and I can confidently say that your body is more than just a medical problem to be solved. It's part of your strength, power, and resilience. That's a beautiful thing.

Understanding your anatomy is key not just to understanding your physical health and communicating with your health team, but it is also a vital part of your emotional health. It helps us feel empowered, confident, and informed when talking about our body. Far too many of us, for far too long, haven't received good, evidence-based information about our anatomy. There is so much power in knowing how your body functions and the purpose of all its parts. What can feel like a big, unmanageable problem can be broken down into what feels like clearer, easy to understand choices.

Now that you are an expert in anatomy, we can delve into some of the more common issues that bring us to the doctor's office. From fibroids and endometriosis to pelvic pain and prolapse, we're going to explore what happens when nature takes a left turn and how you can get your body back on track.

3

Fibroids

My practice is located in New York City, and if you know anything about New York real estate it won't surprise you to hear that my space is very cozy and intimate—translation: small. Every time I exit an exam room and walk back to my office, I pass through the waiting room. It's a quick opportunity to see who is waiting and, let's be honest, to assess how far behind schedule I might be running. One summer afternoon, I noticed a new patient sitting in the chair farthest from the reception desk. As a trained ob-gyn, I can spot a pregnant belly a mile away and she seemed to be almost full term—at least nine months pregnant. The *Price Is Right* was playing on the TV, but she kept her eyes fixed on the ground. About twenty minutes later, I walked into our gynecology exam room—not a room we use for obstetrics—surprised to see her sitting on the table. "Hi, I'm Teresa," she said as she extended her hand to shake mine. I quickly realized she was not pregnant at all, but was someone who needed urgent help with an all too familiar story.

Teresa first complained of heavier periods to her gynecologist when she was twenty-two years old. After a brief evaluation, her doctor told her that she "likely" had fibroids, but did not offer much guidance or follow-up regarding how to diagnose, manage, or treat them. "If they don't bother you, don't bother them" were his parting words of wisdom. Throughout her twenties her periods remained heavy, but she just learned to live and work around them. As she entered her thirties, she noticed that her periods became even heavier and longer—if that was even possible. She talked herself out of seeing another doctor because after several visits, she'd never received any meaningful help. They would tell her that her symptoms just weren't a big deal and were dismissed as just a "normal part of aging."

By her mid-thirties, she started to grow what she described as "a gut." Again, she chalked up her changing body to the typical weight gain associated with age, but her belly continued to grow. It was slow and insidious. She lived in simultaneous fear and denial. Fear of what was going on inside her body and denial that there was in fact something going on inside her body. By this point, Teresa had become what's known in the medical community as a "frequent flier" in her local emergency room. She was known by her name and time of the month, as her heavy bleeding from fibroids routinely brought her in for blood transfusions and pain management.

Teresa saw a few specialists who suggested she have a hysterectomy—the medical term for removal of the uterus—but because she was in her thirties and desperately wanted children, she felt conflicted. Her fibroids continued to grow and began to overwhelm her small frame until she could no longer wear pants and was forced into loose dresses. She soon found that basic movements were becoming painstakingly difficult as the bulge in her belly grew. Bending over, exercise, and even intercourse was no longer comfortable. She felt the life she once loved was slowly slipping away. Teresa was at a crossroads. She was not ready to close the door on children, but she also needed to rescue her declining quality of life.

Teresa's story is, sadly, far too common in my practice. Most women don't just wake up one day and say, "You know what would be fun today, a hysterectomy!" More commonly, the road toward this procedure is like Teresa's—years and years of heavy bleeding interjected by a doctor's visit; a dose of denial; trips to the emergency room for a blood transfusion;

another doctor's visit where your complaints are minimized; years of fertility struggles; ultrasounds; missed work; another dose of denial; a doctor's visit where your only option is a hysterectomy; an ER visit followed by another blood transfusion. This cycle rinses and repeats and before you know it, years have passed. Her journey, like that of hundreds of thousands of other women, is the crossroads of gaps in care and the way women's symptoms, especially gynecological ones, are often overlooked or dismissed.

Let's be real: so many of us have lived with heavy bleeding and pain for so long, we have forgotten what "normal" even looks like, haven't we? Growing up we watched our grandmothers and mothers endure these struggles in silence, and the unspoken expectation was that we, too, must suffer in silence. We saw them miss days of work each month and spend at least the first day of their cycle curled up on the cold bathroom floor, drenched in sweat as waves of cramping pain took over their body. We have internalized these experiences and just thought, "Well, what woman hasn't suffered? Why would I be any different?"

Do you remember when you pieced together your "period survival kit," as your bleeding got worse over time? It started with super tampons. Then you added the overnight pad with wings. Before you knew it you were layering a super tampon, overnight pad, and diaper. *Ugh.* You may have even laid down towels before you went to sleep at night just in case you got your period. Have you ever passed out from bleeding during your cycle or had to visit the ER for a blood transfusion? And do you remember how you felt—physically and emotionally—the first time you passed a blood clot the size of your fist? These moments are more than just inconvenient; they are traumatic.

In my practice, there are two main reasons women opt for a hysterectomy: heavy bleeding and pelvic pain—or sometimes a combination of both. The most common culprit behind heavy bleeding? Uterine fibroids. For pelvic pain, the usual suspects are endometriosis, unsuccessfully treated pelvic inflammatory disease (PID), and adenomyosis. We will tackle endometriosis, its cousin adenomyosis, and PID in the next two chapters but for now we'll take a deep dive into fibroids—the who, why, and what the heck of it all.

The way fibroids impact your life is real. Fibroids disrupt everything from your physical health to your emotional well-being. The ripple effect can be profound. Together, we are going to illuminate everything we know about fibroids—not just for you, but for the generations of women to come after you. Let's get clear about what it means to live with fibroids, and how we can address them head-on.

Uterus Under Siege: A Beginner's Guide to Fibroids

Teresa is not alone in her fibroid struggles and neither are you. Fibroids are by far the most common pelvic complaint in reproductive-age women and the number one reason for hysterectomy in the United States. Studies estimate that 5 to 80 percent of women have fibroids—a staggering range. However, the actual percentage of women who have fibroids could be even higher. Why the uncertainty? Well first of all, many women with fibroids don't experience noticeable symptoms. Second, while we can detect fibroids on ultrasound, diagnosis typically requires surgery, which is the last thing most people want. This gap makes fibroids both under-discussed and underdiagnosed. As a result, many women live without the support or knowledge they need to address the condition effectively.

What Are Fibroids?

I am sure you have heard the word *fibroid* casually tossed around for years—by doctors, family members, friends, and even in pop culture. But what are fibroids, really? The medical term for a fibroid is *leiomyoma*. Let's break that down using some high school Latin:

- *leio* means "smooth"
- *myo* is the root for "muscle"
- *oma* means "tumor" or "growth"

Essentially fibroids are benign smooth muscle tumors. While fewer than one in a thousand fibroids become cancerous, that doesn't mean that they cannot pose serious challenges to your health.

Even with this definition, fibroids might still feel like a mystery. Here is how I explain fibroids to my patients. Fibroids start in the uterus as a single muscle cell—so tiny that you cannot see or feel it. For some reasons we will explore later, this lone cell decides to go rogue and starts growing into a (round) ball of muscle. Some fibroids stop growing when they reach the size of a poppy seed or cherry. Others can be overachievers and grow to the size of a lemon, orange, or even larger sized round, solid ball of muscle.

Fibroids can grow in any zone of the uterus. Remember our papaya analogy?

- **On the outer skin or serosa:** subserosal fibroids.
- **In the juicy flesh or myometrium layer:** intramural fibroids.
- **Just underneath the muscle layer in the center of the uterus:** submucosal fibroids.
- **In the seedy inside or endometrium:** submucosal or intracavitary fibroids.

Any cell in any zone has the potential to transform into a fibroid. Depending on the zone, you may (or may not) have symptoms from your fibroids. Just like real estate, location is everything when it comes to fibroids—location will impact your experience with these tumors. And while some women will only have one or two fibroids over their lifetime, others might carry a tremendous "fibroid burden" with dozens or even hundreds of tumors.

This is why fibroids are so sneaky. Based on how fast they grow, their location in the uterus, and other factors like genetics and environment, some people are overwhelmed with symptoms—bleeding, pain, pressure—while others have none. The size and location of fibroids determine the impact of your symptoms as well as your treatment options, which we discuss in Chapter 5.

Unwitting Poster Child

If fibroids needed a mascot, it would undoubtedly be a Black woman. Armed with a heating pad in one hand and a bottle of ibuprofen in the other, for Black women fibroids are more than just a nuisance. They are a relentless roller coaster of emotional, mental, economic, and physical anguish that we did not sign up for. The numbers speak for themselves: studies show one in four Black women will be diagnosed with fibroids by the age of twenty-five, and this number skyrockets to 80 percent by age fifty. For us, fibroids show up early and often. This means we are more likely to have symptoms earlier in life and are two to three times more likely to have surgery for fibroids compared to white women. This is where knowledge is power and being proactive is key. It is also about being in tune with your body. Knowing what is normal for you and seeking help when something feels off is key to protecting your reproductive health. Women should discuss fibroids with their ob-gyns as early as their twenties and monitor uterine health with regular ultrasounds throughout the thirties and beyond. This way, if you develop fibroids, you can face them head on.

Fibroid Signs and Symptoms

Patients come to my office with a wide range of symptoms, from abnormal bleeding to iron deficiency anemia to chronic pelvic pain and pressure. Some complain of a constant need to urinate as though something is pressing against their bladder, while others complain of constant constipation. Others discover fibroids in the context of infertility or even pregnancy-related complications. In what feels like a twisted game of Would You Rather, fibroids can present with a myriad of frustrating and uncomfortable symptoms. Each person's experience is different, but the disruption is all too real. In the sections that follow, we will dive into the most common symptoms of fibroids, helping you understand what might be causing your discomfort and how these symptoms can be addressed.

Heavy Menstrual Bleeding

For many people with fibroids, heavy bleeding is not just an inconvenience but a life-altering and possibly life-threatening situation. I am not talking about the need for an extra pad or two; I am talking about bleeding so profuse it keeps you running to the bathroom to avoid soaking through your clothing or bedsheets. For people like Teresa, it necessitates trips to the ER because you have become so anemic you can barely function. For many, this type of bleeding doesn't just affect your health—it isolates you. You are trapped at home for days at a time for fear of another embarrassing accident, while the world carries on oblivious to the battle you are secretly fighting.

What Is "Normal," Anyway?

In the United States, most young girls start their periods somewhere between the ages of ten and sixteen years old. Typically, these early periods are light and irregular as the hormonal connection between the brain, ovaries, and uterus is still maturing. This early irregularity is generally not an issue. It is not until you have regular, monthly periods that we get to understand what "normal" looks like for you.

But here is the thing: *normal* is subjective and looks different for everyone. What doctors consider medically "normal" and what you have come to accept as normal may be vastly different experiences.

Medically, a "normal" period is:

- **Duration:** two to seven days of bleeding
- **Frequency:** every twenty-one to thirty-four days, plus or minus a day or two

- **Volume:** about 2.7 ounces, or six tablespoons of blood total—roughly 1.5 shot glasses

As you know your flow can be lighter or heavier throughout the day and week, but on average you should change your pad, tampon, or menstrual cup about every four hours. In general, if you are bleeding for seven or more days, using double or triple protection, or changing more than every four hours then this may be an early sign that something is up. Gynecologists call this heavy bleeding or menorrhagia and it is not something to ignore.

What Causes Heavy Bleeding?

Heavy bleeding can be caused by several conditions, but fibroids are a leading cause. Fibroids in the following locations often contribute to heavy bleeding:

- **Submucosal fibroids:** These grow in or near the endometrium (the uterus's inner lining where menstrual blood originates).
- **Intramural fibroids:** These grow in the myometrium (the uterus's muscular wall).

Fibroids in either of these areas can cause your formerly normal periods to be a nightmare.

The Real Impact of Heavy Bleeding

Over time, your heavy bleeding can have serious consequences for your health. There is a saying in gynecology: *A woman with heavy bleeding is stable—until she isn't.* This means an otherwise young, healthy woman can have months of heavy bleeding and long periods without any issue until suddenly she reaches a tipping point. Blood transports iron, which carries oxygen throughout your body—most importantly to your brain and heart—and is critical to the normal functioning of your body.

Ongoing bleeding leads to anemia—a condition where your body doesn't have enough iron to produce healthy red blood cells. Without enough oxygen, your body can't function properly. Severe anemia can cause:

- Fatigue and weakness
- Fainting or dizziness
- Shortness of breath or chest palpitations
- Cold hands and feet
- In severe cases, chest pain
- At its worst, anemia can land you in the ER. Unfortunately, this is often where I first meet patients suffering from recently diagnosed or undiagnosed fibroids.

Could You Be Anemic?

Even if your periods don't seem unusually heavy, anemia can present in several ways. Ask yourself these questions:

- Do you feel weak and run down?
- Do you have frequent headaches, especially when you are on your period?
- Are you frequently short of breath or have to slow down with the slightest physical exertion?
- Do you feel lightheaded or dizzy?
- Are your hands and feet always cold?

If any of these symptoms sound even remotely familiar, it is worth checking your blood work with basic lab tests. A complete blood count (CBC) and other iron studies can reveal whether your body is running low on fuel. Your symptoms almost always correspond with abnormal results on this blood work. If you have been struggling with these symptoms, listen to your body and reach out to your doctor. There are effective ways to treat your anemia. Treating your anemia can help ward off some of the most taxing symptoms while you are making a solid treatment plan to manage fibroids. When you are not weak, lightheaded, or tired it is much easier to think, make decisions, and regain control over your health and life.

Heaviness and Pressure

Fibroids don't just wreak havoc on your periods—they can also disrupt the delicate balance of your pelvic organs. As fibroids grow, they take up more space in your uterus, which then translates to pressure on nearby structures like your bladder, intestines, and rectum. Think of your pelvis as a tightly packed room with firm walls. When your uterus starts to expand because of fibroids, it essentially crowds out your other organs, forcing them to compete for space. This can lead to a range of frustrating and uncomfortable symptoms like pressure, pelvic heaviness, or discomfort. This pressure can make you constantly feel like you need to urinate frequently and can even cause constipation.

Pelvic Pain

It is true that depending on where your fibroids are located you can also experience a range of pelvic pain symptoms. This pain can range from a dull ache to severe, sharp, and knifelike. When fibroids are positioned on the back side of your uterus, they can put pressure against a complex highway of nerves that run through your pelvic and lower spinal region. These nerves are responsible for sensation and movement in your lower body, including your hip, legs, and feet.

Because of this back-sided pressure, some women report sharp, shooting pain that radiates down one or both legs. It can often be accompanied by numbness, tingling, and a pins-and-needles sensation in the legs or feet. This is much like sciatic pain, which occurs when something like a herniated disc irritates or compresses the sciatic nerve, just this time it is a fibroid. The sciatic nerve is the largest in the body so irritation along its path can create intense and sometimes debilitating pain. If you have ever had sciatic pain, you know this pain is not a joke.

Urinary Symptoms

Fibroids growing outside of the uterus (on the serosa) or in the uterine muscle (intramural fibroids) can create pressure on the bladder leading to a range of urinary symptoms in the same way fibroids can cause pelvic pain. This pressure reduces the space available to fill the bladder and can also interfere with the normal function of the muscles and nerves that control urination. Some of the most common issues include:

- **Weakened urine stream and difficulty emptying the bladder:** As fibroids press against the bladder, you may notice that your once strong stream has become a frustratingly slow dribble. You may also find that sometimes it may feel like you can never fully empty your bladder and you are constantly running to the bathroom. What gives? The pressure of fibroids on your bladder can cause both symptoms. When you cannot totally empty your bladder and hold on to residual urine it creates a perfect environment for bacteria to grow and can increase your risk of recurrent urinary tract infections (UTIs). In more severe cases, large fibroids can even block the urine traveling from your kidneys to your bladder—this can turn your recurrent UTI into a more serious chronic kidney infection.
- **Urinary frequency and urgency:** Fibroids can produce other bladder symptoms, such as frequent trips to the bathroom. When there is pressure on the bladder, the bladder cannot expand as much as it normally would. This means you find yourself having to run to the bathroom much more often to relieve yourself and still you may only pass a small amount of urine each time. Quite frankly, frequent trips to the bathroom can quickly become

annoying as each trip interrupts daily routines and certainly your quality of life.

- **Urinary incontinence:** To layer on another potential complication urinary incontinence or the accidental leak of urine can be a not-so-often talked about but important complication of having fibroids. Even the most minor activities—laughing, sneezing, coughing, exercising—can cause you to leak urine. Sometimes people leak with no specific activity at all. Urinary incontinence happens when the fibroids on the serosa or muscle layer distort the normal pelvic anatomy, which undermines the pelvic floor's ability to support the bladder and urinary tract control mechanisms.

A Growing Belly

Picture this: The uterus can sometimes have a mind of its own and grow to expand outside the pelvis. It may grow so big that it begins to push the boundaries of your pelvis. Very silently, or even sometimes even abruptly your "I'm feeling cute today" outfit now feels tighter and more like, "Why am I carrying this watermelon?" You may even catch your reflection when you walk past a mirror and notice an unexpected lower belly bump, but spoiler alert: this is what we affectionately call a fibroid baby.

This is how it started with my patient Teresa: a slow but steady growth of the uterus that pressed first on the lower and then eventually upper front abdominal muscles. While you may feel pressure internally, physically it may take a little longer before you start to develop a lower belly bulge and look pregnant like Teresa. This moment, my friend, is what I fondly refer to as a "Come to Jesus" moment. Not the kind where lights shine and angels sing, but the kind where your favorite jeans become a bit snug and you are forced to admit that something's up. Even though you were blissfully ignoring your symptoms, a growing belly is really going to grab your attention. Although let's be honest—some people will still brush their symptoms off. I've literally placed a patient's hand right on top of an obvious fibroid-filled uterus, and the patient have told me, "Eh, I just thought I was getting chubby." While fibroids certainly know how to stay under the radar, a growing abdomen is a bright red flag.

And while it may be easy to pretend that it is no big deal, fibroids can literally enter your life like an uninvited roommate. They will rearrange all your furniture, clog your drains, and steal your self-esteem. It is not just about feeling weirdly round in the front of your body, it is how fibroids can make you feel walking throughout life—uncomfortable, self-conscious, and maybe even a little bit hopeless. Trust me, hopelessness is the worst of feelings.

It is my job to help you reclaim their bodies and confidence. I love this part. I'd love it even more if we can pull the brakes on this fibroid train before you're in my office, tearfully wondering if you should start wearing maternity jeans to accommodate your growing belly. That's why early diagnosis and treatment are a big deal. The sooner we catch these uninvited little troublemakers, the sooner you can get back to feeling like *you*. For now, know this: You deserve to feel good in your body, no watermelon belly required.

Fertility under Fire

In most cases—thankfully—fibroids do not interfere with fertility or pregnancy, but there are times where they do. The impact of fibroids on fertility varies from woman to woman. For mothers, fibroids can contribute to pain during pregnancy, increase the risk of Cesarean delivery, as well as the risk for heavy bleeding after delivery, or postpartum hemorrhage. Fibroids can impact the growth of a baby as well as the position of the baby inside the uterus. For some, fibroids can contribute to preterm birth and even first or second trimester miscarriage.

Take Janae, for example. Janae is a patient of mine—young, healthy, and trying to conceive for over four years with her partner. Because she was young, she had been repeatedly reassured to "just keep trying" by other doctors. But every positive pregnancy test ended the same way:

heartache just a few weeks later. When we finally met, I knew we had to dig deeper and be aggressive to help this young couple conceive. A quick round of blood tests and an ultrasound revealed that Janae's uterus had practically become consumed with fibroids.

Janae did know she had fibroids, but was never told they could contribute to infertility. With no other explanation for their fertility struggles popping up, it was time to consider that maybe these unwelcome guests were partly to blame. We developed a plan (which included more imaging and surgery) and got to work, because Janae wasn't ready to give up on building her family—and I wasn't ready to let fibroids call the shots.

Fibroids impact fertility in about 27 percent of women, and in around 3 percent of the time, they can be the sole reason for infertility. We are not entirely sure why these uninvited guests interfere with fertility but there are some solid theories. One idea: Fibroids cause chronic inflammation and/or abnormal blood flow that can interrupt implantation. Other research suggests fibroids can cause contractions that prevent embryos from successful implantation. When submucosal fibroids are present it is thought that they can crowd the cavity of the uterus. Pregnancy and delivery rates are improved when unwelcomed submucosal and intracavitary fibroids are removed.

In Janae's case, her fibroids were very concerning: They were in every location of the uterus. Some were intramural (in the wall of the uterus); some were submucosal (intruding the cavity where the embryo implants); some were serosal and pedunculated. Together, we made a plan that ultimately required surgery to improve her chances of a successful pregnancy. On the day of her surgery I removed forty-two fibroids and reconstructed her uterus. We waited several months as her uterus healed and then she and her husband started trying again. A few months later, she was pregnant, and thirty-seven weeks after that I had the honor of delivering their first baby. Although not everyone's situation is this extreme, the moral of the story is crystal clear: fibroids can have an important impact on fertility. Do not ignore them, and don't let anyone else brush them off either.

* * *

While fibroids may be common, they do not deserve a leading role in your life. Whether they are draining your energy with heavy bleeding, adding pressure where you don't want it, or interfering with your family planning, it is important to be proactive. Take control of your body and health—your fibroids are not the star of the show, you are.

What Causes Fibroids?

I have been asked this question countless times throughout my career, and even after all these years the answer is still lacking. The truth of the matter is that while we know fibroids are essentially overachieving muscle cells that have gone off script, how or why this happens in the first place is still shrouded in scientific, "Huh?"

Here is what scientists have pieced together: there are a lot of moving parts and unanswered questions. There are hormonal, genetic, and environmental components all of which impact the fibroids differently. These factors don't just decide whether fibroids appear; they also influence how they grow, how fast they expand, and how they act once they've taken up residence. But don't lose hope. Understanding these players allows us to craft personalized treatment plans, guiding the hormonal messengers, analyze genetic triggers and address environmental input in a more favorable direction. In other words, while we may not have the full understanding on how fibroids tick, we have a few strategies to explore.

Fibroids, Hormones, and Beyond

Fibroids are unique to women and people with female reproductive hormones. You may have noticed that the stories I have shared so far all include young women—this is because fibroids are the most common tumor among young, reproductive-age women. Hormones play a starring role in the growth of fibroids, and because of that, your hormone story—from when you got your first period to when you hit menopause, and even the use of birth control—can help dictate your fibroid journey and the role they occupy in your body.

To set the scene, there are three primary reproductive hormones: estrogen, progesterone, and testosterone. Of these hormones, estrogen is the headliner that is associated and charged with the stimulation and growth of fibroids. Researchers have found a significant influence of estrogen on fibroids. This hormone attaches to receptors on the fibroid's surface and influences development by sending signals inside the cell that influence growth.

Progesterone, the primary hormone in pregnancy, is also critical in menstruation and influences fibroid growth too. Fibroids are much more likely to form when the hormones estrogen and progesterone are at their highest—hello reproductive years—and are far less likely to form before puberty and during menopause when these hormones are the lowest.

While the research on testosterone and fibroids is limited, there is some evidence to support that high testosterone and estrogen levels may influence fibroids. More research in this area is certainly needed.

Now, your reproductive hormones don't work in isolation. While they may be frontline, we know that there are other proteins that influence fibroid development and growth. Acting along with your reproductive hormones are several well-known proteins called growth factors. You may have never heard these names before, but these proteins do exactly what their name suggests—they make things grow. Much like hormones, they send signals to your cells—in this case the muscle cells of the uterus—to encourage growth. Insulin-like growth factors (IGF), epidermal growth factor (EGF), and transforming growth factor (TGF) are just a few of the proteins that researchers have documented influencing fibroid tumor growth and development. These proteins likely interact with hormones in a cascade of complex physiological processes that contribute to fibroids.

So, what are risk factors you should be aware of? Well, for one thing, if you got your first period early (before ten years of age) your odds of developing fibroids increases. Research also supports changes in our genetics can influence when someone starts their period. This is significant for African American women who, on average, start their periods younger. More specifically, researchers have found eight areas of the genome that are more associated with the age of first period in African American girls. These areas not only influence fibroids, but also overlap with obesity. This is important because obesity (as a high-estrogen state), not only impacts when you get your first period but also fibroids. By identifying women with these genetic markers we can target those at risk for early menstruation and obesity—both of which provide signals to the body impacting fibroid growth.

Hormone exposure is not just about what is happening currently in your body—your mother's hormonal environment while you were in the womb can influence your fibroid risk later on in your life. The infamous drug, diethylstilbestrol (DES) was widely given to pregnant women between 1940 and 1971 to prevent complications during pregnancy. Early exposure to this drug in utero made those babies more susceptible to experiencing their own pregnancy problems, including an increase in fibroids. Thankfully, we've parted ways with DES, but it proves that hormone exposure at any life stage can set the tone for fibroids.

What about modern hormone exposures, like fertility treatments or birth control? Despite what social media myths might tell you, there's no evidence that fertility treatments trigger fibroids; in fact, one large study suggested a *decreased* risk when these treatments work well. And while birth control might seem like a one-way ticket to Fibroid Town (it is a form of hormone exposure, after all), research says otherwise. With millions of women using hormonal fertility treatments each year, this research is reassuring.

The same questions are asked about hormonal birth control. Hormonal birth control has become very controversial, especially in our social media spaces. There are so many myths and misconceptions about what birth control does and does not do to your reproductive system, especially when it comes to fibroids. This in part contradicts everything I just said about hormones contributing to the growth of fibroids. Fortunately for all of us, birth control is one of the most researched aspects of women's health, so let's talk about it!

There's good evidence that hormonal birth control can help manage the heavy bleeding that usually accompanies fibroids, and in some cases can even decrease the size of the tumors. Most hormonal birth control is a combination of a synthetic estrogen and progesterone and some contraceptive options are progesterone only. Synthetic estrogen, or ethinyl estradiol (EE), is the most common estrogen used in birth control and is incorporated into three hundred types of contraceptive oral pills, skin patches, and vaginal insert rings. Like the estrogen your body produces, EE has effects on the ovaries, uterus, and vagina. Unlike the estrogen your body makes, however, EE is more resistant to breakdown in the body making it suitable for long-acting use in medication. It's this quality that allows EE to control fibroids symptoms such as heavy bleeding.

Current research has shown that a moderate (30 to 35 mcg ethinyl estradiol) or low-dose (15 to 20 mcg ethinyl estradiol) daily use does not increase the growth of fibroids. A small, single study, however, suggested that girls who started combined oral contraception between the ages of thirteen to sixteen may have a slight increased risk of fibroids than patients who started at a later age.

Progesterone-only birth control removes estrogen from the equation and is only made with a synthetic version of progesterone—a class of hormones called progestin. Several popular progestin-only contraceptives have been studied in relation to fibroids. The first of these is depo medroxyprogesterone, otherwise known as Depo-Provera or "the shot." It is an intramuscular injection that prevents pregnancy at three-month intervals. It also has been shown to decrease the lining of the uterus making periods very light or absent. Research shows that the use of Depo has been associated with a decrease in bleeding and size of fibroids. This may be helpful for women who present with bleeding and other primary symptoms like pelvic pressure, urinary frequency, and even belly pudge.

Long-acting reversible contraception (LARC) is another widely popular form of progesterone-only contraception. The LARC category includes the progestin-based arm implant and progestin-only T-shaped intrauterine devices or IUDs. While there is strong evidence to suggest that these can help with bleeding related to fibroids, there is limited evidence to suggest that they make fibroids larger or more symptomatic.

The bottom line? Don't let the fear of fibroids steer you away from contraception if you need it. An unplanned pregnancy can be life changing, so concern for both contraception and fibroids is something you and your doctor should balance. With today's data, we can say that balancing your reproductive goals—whether that's preventing pregnancy or managing fibroid symptoms—doesn't have to be a zero-sum game. Stay informed, talk to your doctor, and don't let fibroids call the shots. You should not neglect your reproductive need for contraception because you're afraid that you're going to make your fibroids worse. We don't have any strong evidence to suggest that they will.

Does Pregnancy Influence Fibroid Growth?

When it comes to pregnancy's influence on fibroids, the data is pretty mixed. Some research suggests that having one or more pregnancies after the twenty-week mark may dial down your fibroid risk. Other studies hint that pushing your first birth to a later age could give you a pass from developing fibroids. On the flip side, research also suggests that starting young or spacing your kids far apart might increase your odds of developing fibroids. To make the things even more confusing, there is data to suggest that the more pregnancies you have, the lower your fibroid risk will be.

Admittedly this is all very unclear. The truth is, we don't have the ultimate cheat sheet on how your family-planning timeline affects fibroids. Any advice we may give is basically on a case-by-case basis. Until more conclusive evidence appears, don't treat these early findings as if your fertility journey is set in stone—it is not. Ultimately, the best timing for your family is about what works for you—not what fibroids might prefer. Keep doing what's right for your life, and let the research keep sorting itself out.

Genetics and Lifestyle

Think of your DNA as your body's original blueprint. It sets the stage for how you grow, live, and eventually even gray. Just because your DNA is the universal code for how your body works it does not mean that occasionally the code does not improvise. Lifestyle, environment, and day-to-day choices can influence how our genes turn on and off. Yes, one may have a genetic inclination toward fibroids, but your life and dietary habits and surroundings can influence whether those fibroids take center stage in your reproductive life or wait quietly in the wings.

We've all heard family fibroid tales—grandma, mom, aunts, cousins—passing down not just their fabulous, unaging skin, but also a tradition of fibroid troubles. That's the genetic piece. Typically, these changes are not the action of a single gene, but often several in concert. Chromosomes six, seven, twelve, and fourteen seem to be the major players in fibroid formation but others are possibly involved. Coded in these chromosomes are genes that produce proteins that impact cellular growth and other yet to be understood pathways that contribute to the formation of fibroids. As we move closer to precision medicine and genetic modification, pinpointing these fibroid-linked genes might help us predict (and maybe even prevent!) their growth before they disrupt our health. Until then, think of your genes like the opening credits—they set the tone, but it's your ongoing lifestyle that determines the plot twists.

So yes, your genes can make you more susceptible to fibroids, but this is not the time to feel powerless. You do have some input on determining whether those genes are turned on or off and how they are "transcribed" or "read" by the cells in your body. It has long been known that while genes may lay the foundation for your health or illness, what you put into your body in the form of food, stress, and your environment can influence how these genes manifest in your life. For example, high blood pressure in a family will be different between family members based on the individual—how and what they eat, how often they exercise, where they live, and their level of stress. These modifiable conditions are called social determinants of health and likely impact how fibroids manifest in the lives of women living with them.

Lifestyle, Hormones, and These Crazy Endocrine Disruptors

When it comes to fibroids, hormones definitely play a very important role in how they are expressed in your body. A little discussed caveat, however, is that you and your environment can actually influence your hormones in more ways than you think. Many of the lifestyle habits and practices that put you at greater risk of developing fibroids are those that expose you to chemicals and pollutants that wreak havoc on your hormones. In your body, certain chemicals and pollutants are hormonal impersonators called "endocrine disruptors," which can magnify your already chaotic genetic and hormonal influence on fibroids.

Endocrine (or hormone) disruptors are chemicals that interfere, block, or act like our body's hormones—but not in a good way. Endocrine disruptors act as hormone impersonators that have the master key to the function of your cells and expression of your DNA. They can turn on cell and gene activity without considering the purpose or function of that gene. This lack of discrimination can spark unchecked cell growth and crank up the estrogen dial in your body-setting the stage for several negative side effects in the body, including the growth of fibroids. Endocrine disruptors are found in a wide variety of products in our environment and home. They are present in the plastic ware we use to store food and in the makeup products we routinely use on our skin.

Bisphenol A: The Leading Endocrine Disruptor

Bisphenol A (BPA) is the most famous of these disruptors. BPA lurks in our water bottles, metal food cans, the pesticides used in our food supply, and even in our water supply lines. Everyday plastics, food storage, and food packaging are often our main sources of BPA exposure. So yes, when you are heating up last night's leftovers in a BPA-containing container, you are essentially leaching BPA into your food and ingesting it. BPA has been demonstrated to assist in boosting estrogen levels in the body. BPA has also been found in human fibroid tissue supporting studies that BPA promotes fibroid growth. It has also been linked to activating genes associated with breast cancer. The moral of the story is that BPA should be kept at a distance. Opt for BPA-free packaging and don't heat your food in suspicious plastics.

Phthalates and Parabens

BPA is not the only endocrine disruptor that should be on your radar. The words *phthalates* and *parabens* may have also trickled into your social media feed recently and if they haven't, please listen up. Phthalates make plastic materials longer lasting, more durable, and are also used to dissolve other materials. Sounds pretty innocent until you realize they are found in hundreds of food-packaging products, the vinyl flooring your toddler crawls on, and the personal care products (soaps, shampoos, cosmetics, body washes) that we use every day.

Research tells us that everyone has phthalates in their systems. Large segments of the population have been shown to have these chemicals present in urine testing. Adult women have more exposure than men presumably due to the use of personal care products. African American women have higher rates of exposure than their white counterparts partly due to hair and makeup products as well as environmental and dietary exposures.

Parabens are man-made chemicals that are absorbed through the skin or ingested. They are used as preservatives in makeup, medicine, food, and drinks. The FDA currently allows parabens in packaging as they help products have a longer shelf life and reduce the risk of bacteria and mold in, for example, makeup products. The longer the chemical tail structure of parabens, the more they act like estrogen, nudging your body to respond to its estrogenlike signals. Parabens were once labeled as harmless, but now we know that parabens disrupt the normal functioning of both male and female reproductive functioning, development, and fertility. Parabens have been linked to the development of skin irritations, breast cancer, and you guessed it, fibroids.

Watch Those Labels!

The take-home message is to check the labels on your food, health, and beauty products. Words ending in -*paraben* such as *butylparaben, isobutylparaben, butylparaben, isopropylparaben*, and *propylparaben* are red flags. Similar to anything with the word *phthalate* in it, such as *butyl benzyl phthalate, dibutyl phthalate*, or *diethyl phthalate*. Now many products proudly flaunt labels like "paraben free" and "phthalate free." Your reproductive system depends on you to make informed decisions so—as best as possible—build your life around BPA-, paraben-, and phthalate-free materials. Your uterus will thank you.

Other Lifestyle Modifications

Avoiding phthalates and parabens is one step to take. Here are some other changes you can make to improve your symptoms.

- **Red meat:** Research supports that diets high in red meat are more associated with an increased risk of diabetes and cardiovascular disease versus plant-based diets. It should not come as a surprise to learn that diets high in beef and other red meats and ham also have a respective 1.7 and 1.3-fold increase relative risk of fibroids.

- **Alcohol:** Consumption of alcohol, especially beer, appears to be associated with an increased risk of developing fibroids.
- **Smoking:** There is a bit of a head-scratcher here as there is some conflicting research in this area. Some research suggests that smokers may have a slightly lower risk of fibroids—gasp! It is thought that the chemical in cigarette smoke may interfere with a key enzyme called aromatase that is used to make estrogen. Now, this doesn't give you permission to pick up a pack of cigarettes just to keep fibroids at bay. No other studies have supported these limited results, and we have mountains of evidence showing smoking is harmful in every other aspect of your health. In essence, don't even think about lighting up for the sake of fewer fibroids.

Social and Environmental Risks

It is no secret that fibroids play favorites when it comes to ethnic groups, showing up much earlier, growing faster, and causing more severe problems in women of African descent when compared to white women. It is not, however, the melanin alone that sets these differences in health-related experiences into motion. It is the social and environmental realities often tied to race—such as unequal access to healthcare, chronic exposure to certain pollutants, and the relentless toll of racism—that leave their fingerprints all over this disparity.

In other words, what looks like a race-based difference in fibroid development is really an impact of the social determinants of health. Social determinants of health are the everyday conditions in which people live, work, and play. They shape everything from diet and exercise opportunities to stress levels, neighborhood environments, and exposure to harmful chemicals. All of these factors can turn certain genes on or off—like flipping molecular switches—and influence how the body grows and manages fibroids.

One of the most insidious social determinants of health is stress. Chronic stress, especially fueled by discrimination and social disadvantage, has the power to reach deep into our genetic machinery and only recently is this phenomenon getting the research attention it deserves. Over time, unrelenting stress from racism, slavery, poverty, war, and other events can influence how DNA is read and translated by the body's cells. This can mean that fibroid-related genes may be activated or intensified under certain high-stress conditions, leading to more pronounced symptoms and tougher outcomes.

The upside of discussing and researching the impact of social determinants of health is we are finally addressing fibroid disparities beyond one's individual biology. It calls for recognizing that who gets fibroids—and how severely they experience them—has roots in long-standing social inequities. It means a multipronged strategy to help close this environmental stress gap, including increased access to healthier foods (like fruits and vegetables); combating exposure to environmental toxins (BPA, parabens, and phthalates); and reducing chronic stress through community support, health policy changes, and improved access to care. The hope is that by tackling the social and environmental stressors that may trigger fibroids, we can dial back fibroid rates in the most affected communities and improve women's health across the board.

Chew on This:
Nutrition That May Keep Fibroids at Bay

You might not be surprised to learn that loading up on fruits and vegetables (especially citrus fruit) could slightly reduce your risk of fibroids, but who knew that a latte or a scoop of ice cream might also help keep fibroids at bay? This interesting plot twist is supported by the Black Women's Health Study, which aimed to identify what Black women can do to decrease the risk of uterine fibroids. In this study, increased dairy intake—whether full or low fat—was suggested to help lower fibroid risk. This flips theories on dairy's reputation as being inflammatory.

While more research is needed, it is possible that the actual benefit may come from calcium or even vitamin D—both of which are heavily present in dairy. The role of vitamin D is especially important for people with deeper skin tones who tend to have lower vitamin D levels. Since Black women in the US generally consume less dairy, increasing their intake and ensuring adequate vitamin D might help explain and possibly reduce some of the environmentally based differences we see in fibroid rates.

Bottom line: A little more milk and a bump in vitamin D might help keep fibroids off the menu. It's not a miracle cure, but certainly worth more definitive research.

* * *

You may be a little annoyed by the unlucky genetic draw to have inherited this fibroid burden—but do not lose heart. Your fate is not sealed. By knowing how fibroids take shape, where they live and how they can behave you'll be better equipped to keep them in check. After all, understanding the enemy is half the battle—and by now you understand her really well.

Armed with this knowledge, you can walk into your doctor's office, ready to weigh the pros and cons of every option, but before you even get there you will have already transitioned your diet to one that is primary plant-based (or at least lower in red meat) and have also considered starting a calcium and vitamin D supplement. This is you taking the reins and moving forward to the health and wellness you deserve.

4

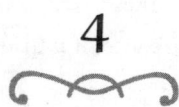

Pelvic Pain

Endometriosis and Adenomyosis

When it comes to reasons women feel ready to evict their uteruses, pelvic pain is a major offender—right up there with fibroids. *Pelvic pain* is the deceptively simple, catchall term for the number of ways we experience full-on, life-disrupting pain in our lower body. It is not just a little twinge or discomfort, but a life-changing, all-consuming total body experience that can take over your entire life. Chronic pelvic pain, defined as pain lasting more than six months, affects 14 to 32 percent of women worldwide. For about one-third of people, the pain gets so intense that it forces them to cancel work, slashes income, and steals the joy from their daily lives. It is no wonder that pelvic pain is the second-most common reason women choose to have a hysterectomy.

The main culprit behind much of our pelvic pain is endometriosis, a complicated inflammatory condition that can be challenging to diagnose and treat, and its cousin adenomyosis. But before we zero in on endometriosis we must look at the bigger picture of how pelvic pain can lead to you wanting a hysterectomy. Your pelvis is a complex neighborhood of organs, muscles, connective tissue, and nerves—any of which can stir up trouble. For this reason, it is helpful to take a bird's-eye view of other conditions that can cause pain before we lump everything in an "endometriosis" box. As we aim to understand the cast of characters in your pelvis, you give yourself a clear understanding as to what may be happening. Rarely do any of these symptoms happen in isolation. The goal is not to just identify the cause, it is also to achieve relief.

The Many Faces of Pelvic Pain: Thinking Holistically About Your Pelvis

Your pelvis is the body's version of an everything bagel: this small, compact, bony structure has several systems running through it. Your pelvis helps you walk, stand, and basically perform every movement you can consider. Your internal pelvic structures host everything from your reproductive organs (uterus, fallopian tubes, and ovaries), digestive system (intestines and rectum), urinary system (bladder and ureters), as well as a complex basket of interwoven muscles, nerves, and blood vessels. Almost every system of your body is represented in the pelvis, tightly packed and intimately touching the next system—like an everything bagel. It makes sense that when something is off it can really set the entire area into a spiral.

With so many "systems" in your pelvis it can take time, patience, imaging, and sometimes even surgery before we can figure out what is going on. When a patient comes into my office and says, "I have pelvic pain," my first thought is "Okay, where exactly?" We need to slow down and dig in to figure out where the root of your discomfort lies. With so many potential suspects, often my first question is, "How do you describe your pain?" Is it sharp or dull? Is your pain primarily in one location or does it move from one side of the body to the next? Is it primarily in your abdomen or does it travel, shooting down the back of your lower back and legs. Is it persistent or does it throb for hours before it goes away? Does it go away without or without pain medication?

As women, we often look at pelvic pain and assume it must be our uterus or some other reproductive part that is causing trouble. This line of thinking can often misdirect you and delay proper treatment. Yes, chronic pelvic pain can absolutely start in your reproductive organs with medical conditions like endometriosis, but the real villain could very well be a fussy bladder or chronic constipation. This is why taking a holistic, all-hands-on-deck approach is important for you. It means you and your medical team will not assume we know what is wrong or ignore the other potential culprits in your pelvis—in this way we will not offer you a hysterectomy for what might actually be a bladder problem, constipation, or even bad posture. You see, the pelvis is amazingly interconnected. We need to consider each system both individually and as part of the larger picture. This is how we approach pelvic pain holistically.

Muscles in Action: The Unsung Heroes of the Pelvic Floor

Let's just say that motherhood will never cease to keep you humble and remind you who is boss. I was reminded of the hidden power of the pelvic floor almost immediately after delivering my first baby. After pushing out an eight-pound, three-ounce baby in just under twenty minutes, I felt like my pelvis had staged a complete mutiny. Everything—and I mean everything—was on fire. Most of the time I needed help with even the simplest of movements. Getting in and out of bed, sitting down, and even walking felt like a Herculean task. My entire pelvis felt like it was going to fall out. It was unlike anything I had ever experienced.

Then came my real wake-up call. One morning, while my husband was helping me get out of bed, he cracked a little joke about the baby that was just funny enough I let out a small laugh. Before I knew it (and to my absolute horror), I felt warm water travel down my leg, instantly soaking through my underwear and pj's, splashing onto the wood floor and covering my husband's sock-covered feet like someone had dropped a water balloon. My full bladder decided to empty itself without so much as a warning or a heads-up. The truth hit me right then: my pelvic floor, a set of muscles I took for granted and rarely ever considered, was now running the show and I had some serious catching up to do to heal it.

That was my first wake-up call, but it wasn't the last. Honestly, for several years after birth, it seemed to hold a grudge against me—letting loose a little surprise when I coughed or sneezed, jumped rope, or even stood up too fast. My disrespectful pelvic floor would rear her head at the most inconvenient times. Eventually, panty liners became my everyday armor, warding off any embarrassing "waterworks" at the office. This experience taught me a tough lesson—we never appreciate our pelvic floor until it stages a full-blown protest.

Your pelvic floor muscles are like a hammock that hangs from your pelvic and hip bones and wraps from the front to the back of your body, allowing for normal bodily function. They are the gatekeepers to holding it all together—pee, poop, and even sex. When one or all of these muscles fail, life can get a little messy, and even wet. These muscles can be tight, loose, weak, or a combination of all three. Add in any scar tissue from birth, as well as other physical and emotional trauma, then you have got yourself a complex support system in dire need of attention. When these muscular gatekeepers falter, words like *accident, messy,* and *bathroom* become a regular part of your vocabulary.

The MVP of your pelvic support team is your levator ani muscle. As the name implies, like an elevator, the levator ani lifts and supports the organs. The powerhouse is not just one big muscle, but actually three muscles working together from the front of your body at the pubic symphysis stretching all the way back to your tailbone. One of the key muscles, the pubococcygeus, controls both the flow of urine and the contractions of your pelvis during an orgasm. Meanwhile, a smaller, triangle-shaped muscle called the coccygeus joins with your levator ani to complete what we call your pelvic floor. Together, they hold down the fort, making sure your pelvis organs stay where they should.

Like any other muscle in your body, your pelvic floor can become fatigued, stressed, overworked, and start to ache. Nerves can become irritated, and the surrounding connective tissue inflamed creating a snowball effect of irritation, inflammation, and eventually pain. After several weeks to months of chronic stress on these muscles you can start to have pelvic floor dysfunction.

There are several sources of pelvic floor stress that can lead to pelvic floor dysfunction. The reason for the stress and how it contributes to chronic pelvic pain may (or may not) influence your decision to have a hysterectomy:

- **Pregnancy and childbirth:** It is not surprising that carrying around a growing baby for ten months can give your pelvic floor a serious workout. Each pregnancy adds more strain, leaving your muscles compromised. Hours of pushing, vaginal lacerations, and even Cesarean birth can take their toll on your pelvic floor.
- **Obesity:** Extra pounds aren't just tough on your knees; they can also give your pelvic floor a rough ride. Over time, excess weight turns into constant downward pressure on those muscles eventually causing an internal heavy, achy feeling inside. It is just a reminder that excess weight weighs on your pelvic floor more than you think and maintaining a regular weight is helpful to keep her healthy.
- **Chronic cough:** Who knew a little cough could do so much damage? Well, your pelvic floor knows. While it may seem harmless, each "ahem" sends repeated tiny pressure to your pelvic floor. Over time, these micro stresses can accumulate, weakening your pelvic floor muscles and leaving you feeling heavy and weighed down.
- **Constipation:** While constipation may seem innocent enough, chronic straining to move your bowels is a similar stress to carrying a baby or that never-ending cough. Forcing those muscles to do heavy lifting in the bathroom will eventually tire them out, leaving them weaker and less supportive over time.
- **Hormonal shifts:** As estrogen wanes during menopause, your pelvic floor can notice a decline in elasticity, strength, and tone

making it more challenging to keep your internal organs in place. While it may be slow and subtle, things may start to slowly shift downward—a perfect setup for pelvic organ prolapse.

- **Trauma:** Trauma is not just "in your head." It can leave physical and emotional fingerprints on your pelvic floor causing chronic pelvic pain. In some cases, your pelvic floor muscles can clamp down in a condition known as vaginismus. Survivors of physical or sexual trauma often have their pelvic pain overlooked and misdiagnosed.
- **Endometriosis:** Conditions like endometriosis (see below) and fibroids (see Chapter 3) can also weigh on and inflame the pelvic floor.
- **Bladder dysfunction:** Conditions that cause pain or stress on your bladder can also contribute to pelvic floor dysfunction. Frequently holding in your urine, recurrent urinary tract infections, and bladder pain syndrome (formerly known as interstitial cystitis) can lead to pain and inflammation which, over time, can injure your pelvic floor.
- **Infection:** Pelvic pain can also be caused by infections such as chlamydia, gonorrhea, syphilis, HIV/AIDS, trichomoniasis, vaginitis, and also genital herpes. If untreated or if treatment is delayed, inflammation can spread across the pelvic floor and lead to recurrent pain.

When you think of how common conditions such as pregnancy, obesity, and constipation are, it's no wonder that so many women experience pelvic pain. There is good news—you are not stuck with being "uncomfortable" for your entire life. The first step is to have a heart-to-heart with your doctor about your pelvic pain and discomfort. It is important to rule out any medical conditions that may contribute to your pelvic floor dysfunction. It might be as simple as improving your diet or adding a stool softener to alleviate chronic constipation. Most importantly, do not hesitate to discuss a referral to a pelvic physical therapist. A pelvic physical therapist is a personal trainer for your pelvic floor. Their role in your pelvic floor health cannot be underestimated. A pelvic PT is trained to figure out which muscles are tight, weak, spastic, and then coach them back into normal shape. They will help you learn exercises, stretches, and techniques to help your pelvic floor get its groove back. For you this means an end to your pain, fewer leaks, and a happier life below the belt.

Bladders Behaving Badly

Bladders can be real troublemakers. Sometimes it is the bladder alone staging a protest and in other cases there can be an overlap in pelvic floor dysfunction and bladder symptoms. Bladder pain most commonly occurs during urination. When we urinate, the muscles of the bladder contract to move urine out of the bladder and through the urethra. There are some medical conditions that can make this emptying movement uncomfortable:

- **Recurrent urinary tract infections (UTIs):** Some culprits to urinary pain are well known, like a UTI. UTIs happen when bacteria repeatedly enter your bladder and turn the urethra and bladder lining into a red, inflamed battle ground. UTIs present with a range of symptoms, like blood in your urine, having to go to the bathroom frequently (urinary urgency), or feeling like you have to urinate, but nothing comes out (hesitancy). Most classically, a UTI cannot only cause discomfort, but make you feel like you are urinating pure fire (dysuria). Recurrent UTIs mean you experience three or more UTIs in a year. This is the case for approximately 20 to 40 percent of women. When you are dealing with recurrent UTIs it can leave your bladder in a constant state of inflammation and eventually lead to chronic bladder pain even when you don't have an active infection.

- **Interstitial cystitis (IC):** IC—now called bladder pain syndrome (BPS)—is the wild card in the world of pelvic pain. IC/BPS is not caused by a bacteria or virus we can pinpoint, but some other yet unknown cause that makes a red and angry bladder send pain signals to the lower abdomen, urethra, and even the vagina. IC/BPS can seem like a UTI with extreme pain and frequent urination. You may use the bathroom more than you thought possible—upward of sixty times a day.

Yet even with what we do know, we are not sure what causes IC/BPS other than it is more common in women. Could it be an autoimmune disorder, an allergy, or some mysterious trigger we haven't discovered yet? Until we figure it out, IC/BPS remains a diagnosis of exclusion, meaning we should test for everything else first—infection, nerves, allergies—and rule them all out before saying, "Yep, this pelvic pain is because of IC/BPS."

Urine Incontinence

Think of your bladder like that unreliable friend who bails at the worst times. One moment you're mid-laugh, mid-cough, or mid-burpee, and bam—your bladder decides it's showtime. That's what we call stress incontinence. Then there's the drama queen version: your bladder says "Go! Go! Go!" and you sprint to the bathroom, only to find you have hardly any urine to show for it. Five minutes later, same drill. That's urge incontinence, also known as an overactive bladder, or OAB.

Unfortunately, these symptoms do not necessarily mellow with age. As we get older, our bladders can become as dramatic as a telenovela. Foods and drinks that once treated you kindly now leave your bladder doing the cha-cha at any moment. Well-known bladder stimulants such as caffeine, mint, chocolate, citrus, or too much liquid, especially carbonated water, can stress your bladder out. And while sure, peeing every two seconds may not cause full-blown chronic pelvic pain, your bladder and pelvic floor are neighbors that need to live in harmony. Sometimes making a few dietary and lifestyle tweaks can help quiet the bladder drama and keep the pelvic floor peace.

The Vulva

You may think the vulva is quietly tucked away as the entrance to the vagina, but it's actually got quite an intense nerve network connecting to not only your spine, but also to your pelvic floor. With so much sensory real estate, trouble can easily present itself. Pain from the vulva is more common than you think, affecting about two hundred thousand women every year. Remember that your vulva includes the labia (major and minora), the vaginal opening, the clitoris, and the vestibule. The nerves that innervate this area start at your lower spine and stretch down into your pelvis and settle in the vulva, clitoris, and rectum. That's a massive potential area of pain.

Vulvar pain can stem from infection (yeast or herpes infections); nerve injury (nerve compression or trauma); cancer (squamous skin cancer); inflammation (lichen sclerosus); trauma (vaginal birth, use of forceps, sexual assault); low estrogen states (menopause or breastfeeding); and even radiation or chemotherapy. Sometimes we can't identify any particular reason why you're experiencing vulvar pain. In this case we call it vulvodynia, especially when the pain lasts for three or more months. Vulvar pain can come and go, or be triggered by sex, tampons, toilet tissue, or simply sitting down for too long. Vulvar pain can throb, burn, or sting—like when you pour alcohol on a cut. It can be painful and make daily activities like wearing underwear or tight clothing unbearable.

Over time, constant pain signals from your vulva keep your pelvic floor tense and contracted. This can make pelvic muscles tired, weak, and unable to function properly. Like constipation, painful sex, or urinary retention, vulvar pain can contribute to pelvic floor dysfunction. So, while you may not notice this happening, this vicious cycle can lead to discomfort that has to be addressed before it takes over your life.

The Proximity of It All

Your pelvis is an important part of your daily life and, as you can see, an amazingly complex area of your body. Dealing with pelvic pain is like living with several roommates in a cramped one-bedroom apartment. Who knows what is acting up at any given time in these tight quarters. The uterus? The bladder? The rectum? The pelvic floor nerves and muscle? Or maybe it's a little pettiness from everyone. This is why it is important to keep a wide focus on pelvic pain and seek a multispecialty approach before assuming it is the uterus and making an irreversible decision to remove it without a thorough investigation.

Endometriosis: Finally Getting You the Attention You Deserve

Endometriosis is having a moment, and it's about time, if you ask me. Back in my medical school and residency days, it was basically a mythical creature. If you brought it up, you might get a few raised eyebrows from one or two professors, but discussions about endometriosis were few and far between. But oddly enough, if you flip through older medical texts, surprise, surprise, you will see concepts of endometriosis peeking through the pages as early as the 1700s. By 1860, pathologists had already connected the dots between the symptoms of endometriosis with microscopic evidence of the disease. Yet here we are, still leaving patients in limbo for an average of seven years before anyone says, "Yes, this is real. You are not imagining your symptoms." I have met patients who have searched upward of twenty years for answers while other patients never receive a clear diagnosis or treatment.

Let me introduce you to Vanessa, one of those patients. She carried her entire medical history in a notebook when she came to see me, traveling from Delaware to New York with a stack of imaging studies, previous doctors' notes, and a pharmacist's dream list of medications that never did the trick. Her journal detailed menstrual pain starting as early as thirteen where she would curl up on the bathroom floor, missing out on school, time with friends, and basically her childhood. For decades she'd tried everything—pain meds, birth control, and a parade of specialists including pain management, ob-gyns, urologists, gastroenterologists, and even psychologists. Still, no answers.

Over her lifetime she had tried over twenty treatments for her pain and despite all this, no one could tell her what was causing her relentless pain and subsequent depression. After decades of training and then caring for women like Vanessa, I have come to learn there are only a handful of conditions that are as absolutely consuming as endometriosis. I sent her for a series of tests including an MRI and an ultrasound. When I told her I suspected endometriosis had likely spread throughout her pelvis she cried tears of relief. Simply hearing the word *endometriosis* was affirming for her. "I knew I wasn't making it all up," she said. Having her pain acknowledged as real and worthy of a name was as healing as the diagnosis itself.

What Is Endometriosis?

Endometriosis, fondly nicknamed "endo," is when the endometrium, the specialized lining of the uterus, goes rogue in your pelvis. Instead of shedding every month and exiting the body, the endometrium packs up its bags and moves to other parts of your reproductive system, and even sometimes well beyond. Once the endometrial tissue settles outside of your uterus it continues to function like endometrium; it makes blood and causes chronic inflammation and scar tissue because it is in an area it does not belong. This inflammation and scar tissue then lead to heavy, painful periods, stubborn pelvic pain, fertility roadblocks, and much, much more.

About 5 to 10 percent of reproductive-age women in the United States are battling endometriosis. That is upward of 6.5 million women— enough to fill a few major cities—and that figure is likely an underestimate since endometriosis is notoriously underdiagnosed. Given the potential impact on your life, endometriosis is a diagnosis that we cannot afford to miss.

Rethinking Endometriosis:
Breaking the "White Woman Only" Stereotype

In the summer of 1939, Dr. Joe Vincent Meigs penned one of the earliest op-eds on what we now know as endometriosis. While he offered valuable clinical insight, let's just say his social commentary should have come with a trigger warning. As you can imagine, his views were dripping with the patriarchal and racist tropes that—you guessed it—helped shape the minds of generations of doctors learning about endometriosis at that time and even today.

In essence, Meigs believed that endometriosis was increasing because women were having children later in life. His remedy? Marry young, procreate early and often, and then, after you've popped out a few kids, feel free to use birth control. Well, okay maybe those were not his exact words…here are his exact words: "It is better for us, as doctors and fathers, to urge early marriage and early and frequent childbearing." He said "young married couples should be urged to have children early, and practice contraception after they have their families. They should be taught how to have children, not avoid them."

That's right—he said get hitched, have babies, and everything will be just fine…Well sure, only if our uterus and endometriosis got the memo about our perfectly planned timeline.

He also framed endometriosis as a disease of the "well-to-do" women, which in 1939 was code for affluent and white. This laid the foundation for the stereotype that persists to this very day that endometriosis is a white woman's disease. Later researchers leaned in, painting endometriosis patients (in predominantly white research studies) as "well dressed with trim figures," intensely driven, and ambitious, because these qualities were—according to them—somehow risk factors for pelvic pain. So while the face of fibroids may be a Black woman, thanks to these accounts from the 1930s, the poster child for endometriosis solidly became an overachieving, goal-oriented, perfectionist white woman—particularly those who are "married to men who are equally well-educated, highly motivated, and achievement-oriented."

Now this is not just some weird, anecdotal historical foot-note. This and other stereotypes have real consequences. They reinforce racial bias in medicine and impact how endometri-osis is diagnosed and treated—even decades later. Doctors have been trained, often unconsciously, to see endometriosis as a dis-ease of white, upper-class women, leaving other people, i.e., poor, non-white, nonheterosexual people, who have historically have complaints of pelvic pain overlooked or dismissed further written out of the medical literature. This manifests as studies demonstrating that Black women often wait longer for diagno-sis and treatment, meaning painful life-altering symptoms go unaddressed.

We must call out these old, biased narratives for what they are: outdated tropes that continue to uphold racism and patri-archy in medicine and keep countless people from getting the care they deserve. As anyone with endometriosis will tell you: endometriosis does not care about your ethnicity, gender orien-tation, bank account, or wardrobe, so neither should medicine.

Why Does the Endometrium Go Rogue?

The truth is, after all these years we are not entirely sure why endometri-osis happens, but there are some helpful theories to consider. The most popular theory is called "retrograde menstruation," which happens because some menstrual blood moves backward through your fallopian tubes and into your pelvis instead of flowing out through the vagina. The backward flow of blood may be encouraged by uterine contractions pushing the blood in the wrong direction or perhaps due to a blockage like a closed hymen or a closed cervix.

Retrograde menstruation is pretty common—over three-quarters of women with open fallopian tubes have period blood that moves backward into their pelvis when they menstruate. This back-flowing menstrual blood comes into contact with the ovaries, fallopian tubes, lower pelvis, rectum, and the uterosacral ligaments—common sites for endometriosis to implant. Despite how common this is, not all of these women will develop endometriosis. We believe it is because endometriosis is more complicated than this. We can only speculate that some women may have a genetic predisposition to developing endometriosis. When a genetic risk combines with hormonal factors, it leads to a perfect storm for developing endometriosis at these sites.

We can also consider the metaplasia theory. This is the idea that endometriosis does not start from the rogue, backward movement of blood but instead starts in normal (stem) cells already present in the abdomen. This theory suggests that stem cells can transform into endometrial cells when hormones like estrogen and other genetic and immunological factors help initiate this change. Unfortunately, the exact who, what, and why of hormones and immune factors has still yet to be discovered, but this idea helps explain why some young women without retrograde menstruation develop endometriosis.

There is even research to suggest that endometrial cells can travel from the uterus to other locations in your body via the blood or lymphatic system. It is also possible that in rare cases direct transplantation of endometrial cells to other locations in the pelvis can happen after surgery, like a C-section or even hysterectomy. All in all, endometriosis is crafty, and we are still piecing together the puzzle of how it sets up shop where it does not belong.

Not a One-Size-Fits-All Condition

Endometriosis can look very different for everyone, and the severity of the disease can vary widely in two primary ways. The first is infiltration, or how deeply the endometrial tissue dives down or tunnels into healthy tissue. Eighty percent of women have superficial endometriosis, which involves shallow implants, or patches of endometrial tissue, developing on the surface of organs (bladder, rectum, ovaries, et cetera). While these implants cause inflammation leading to your painful symptoms, they have not penetrated the tissues too deeply. About 1 to 5 percent of women experience deep infiltration. Deep infiltration means endometrial tissue burrows beyond the superficial or top layers of the organs. While this is a smaller percentage of endometriosis the damage is more significant. Deep lesions often lead to thickened tissue and scars forming between your organs. You might develop more severe symptoms as a result, making treatment more challenging.

In addition to superficial and deep infiltration, you must also think about how far beyond your uterus endometriosis has spread. To make sense of all this, we rely on four stages, with stage 1 being when the endometrial patches are mostly small, superficial, and located only in or near your pelvic organs, and stage 4 representing a full-blown takeover of endometriotic implants both near and beyond the pelvis. Let's break it down:

- **Stage 1—Minimal.** This is when small, very superficial endometrial implants are on or near your pelvic organs and can be easily removed during surgery. In stage 1, there is no scar tissue causing the organs to stick together.
- **Stage 2—Mild.** In stage 2 there are more implants in the pelvis and endometriosis is found on the ovary. The implants are not deeply invasive and can still be surgically removed and no significant scar tissue is present.
- **Stage 3—Moderate.** This moderate stage of disease is hallmarked by multiple deep and superficial implants all over the pelvis. Your

reproductive anatomy is distorted and starts to stick to each other due to scar tissue. In stage 3, one or both ovaries are affected by or endometriomas—endometrial blood-filled cysts that have the appearance and texture of milk chocolate when opened, or "chocolate cysts."

- **Stage 4—Severe.** In this more advanced stage, both deep and superficial lesions are all over the pelvis. The associated scar tissue and inflammation can involve your uterus, fallopian tubes, ovaries, and even rectum. This can affect your fertility by causing the organs to stick together and distort your normal anatomy.

While there is not technically a stage 5, in a rare subset of women, sometimes endometriosis can be more aggressive, traveling beyond the pelvis to locations like the skin, lungs, intestines, or even the brain. Just remember, these stages typically only get confirmed once a surgeon takes a peek inside your abdomen during an operation. If you head to the operating room for treatment, such as a hysterectomy, expect your doctor to take notes on how far endometriosis has spread and this may impact your treatment plan after surgery.

Symptoms of Endometriosis

Endometriosis is more than just a nasty, painful period. You would be mistaken to minimize endometriosis pain to a few days of the month. Endometriosis is a chronic condition that follows you throughout your entire reproductive years impacting every cycle, every relationship, your thoughts about your career and family planning, even your sanity causing profound depression and anxiety. Imagine being sidelined by relentless pain or fatigued by a body that seems to be working against your every desire to grow your family, or even simply feel normal. For some, endometriosis may be period pain that laughs at over-the-counter painkillers and sends you straight to the ER for stronger stuff. For some, it is not just killer cramps, but also painful sex, digestive trouble, or the constant emotional whiplash of not knowing how you will feel on a day-to-day basis. These symptoms, though common among those with endometriosis, are unfortunately dismissed or misunderstood. Let's take a closer look at what endometriosis might feel like and how it can impact day-to-day life to help you connect the dots and find the support you need.

Painful Periods

Pain is a common and debilitating symptom of endometriosis. We all know that periods can be painful, but for folks with endometriosis, the pain is on another level. In fact, painful periods, also known as dysmenorrhea, can be so intense it can rival childbirth or passing a kidney stone. Ibuprofen or other over-the-counter pain medication, might as well be a breath mint when it comes to endometriosis pain. After so many years of dealing with painful periods, you often quickly pivot to the emergency room for much stronger pain medication because nothing else will help.

The type of pain may vary as well. It can take the form of gut-wrenching spasms that prevent you from getting out of bed. You may experience a dull, throbbing pressure in your belly that makes it feel like your uterus is going to fall out of your vagina. Some describe a twisting internal sensation as if someone is wringing out their uterus like wet laundry. You may also describe sharp, knifelike pain that shoots down your abdomen, back, vagina, bladder, and rectum. Some people even faint from the sheer intensity of pain. This is not a sustainable way of life.

Heavy Periods

If that wasn't enough, endometriosis can come with heavy menstrual bleeding, also known as menorrhagia. If you have heavy bleeding, we should also consider adenomyosis, which I describe as a close cousin to endometriosis. Adenomyosis occurs when endometrial cells burrow into the uterine muscle itself. This causes the walls of the muscle to swell and inflame. Adenomyosis is a double whammy because not only are your periods painful, but they are also heavy. Like endometriosis, adenomyosis is still poorly understood, but we know it can occur after surgeries like C-sections or perhaps by the reverse flow or retrograde menstruation.

Painful Intercourse

Pain during sex is another big, red flag. Also known as dyspareunia, painful intercourse can feel like a sharp, stabbing sensation, deep aches, or even an internal burning sensation regardless of your partner, timing, or sexual position. Discussing sex and intimacy might feel embarrassing with your care providers, but it is very important. Pain with sex is not normal and endo can turn intimacy into a nightmare.

The type of pain you experience can help suggest where the lesions in your body may be. Superficial pain happens at the entrance of the vagina when you try to insert anything into the vagina. This can happen with implants on the hymen, perineum, or on the cervix. On the other end of the spectrum, if you have endometrial tissue in your uterus, back vaginal wall, or on the front of your rectum, sexual pain can be felt deep inside your pelvic organs during penetration.

So remember that you are not imagining the pain or discomfort, nor should you sweep it under the rug. Pain with sex is real and endometriosis might be the culprit.

Chocolate Ovarian Cysts

Ovarian cysts—fluid-filled sacs in the ovary—are very commonplace in gynecology and generally nothing to worry about. The fluid inside often gets reabsorbed over time and does not require surgery. In endometriosis, these cysts are called "chocolate cysts" or endometriomas because they are lined with endometrium which produces a thick, brown liquid that looks like melted chocolate. Finding an endometrioma is a major first sign of endometriosis. The inflammatory fluid inside the chocolate cysts can cause the ovaries, fallopian tubes, and uterus to stick together.

In rare cases—typically less than 0.8 percent—endometriomas can become cancerous. This should be considered if you are over forty-five or if you have large cysts (nine centimeters or bigger). Endometriomas that are large and have an abnormal appearance should be removed. If you have a family history of ovarian cancer, a cyst that is getting bigger, or if your ultrasound or MRI that demonstrates features of cancer, you should talk with your doctor about next steps which will likely involve surgery.

Gastrointestinal Discomfort

Just like sex, no one ever likes to talk about poop, even though everyone does it. Recently, a new endometriosis patient of mine came in, hands in the air, exasperated, saying "It's the poop! Why doesn't anyone talk about the poop?" I happily obliged because, yes poop matters, especially with endometriosis. Somewhere between 5 to 25 percent of women with endo experience significant gastrointestinal symptoms, but you'd never know it because it's not often discussed.

Endometriosis in the gastrointestinal system is sneaky, and symptoms emerge when endometriosis implants on the intestines, colon, or rectum. This creates the sensation of sharp shooting pain throughout your stomach and lower abdomen. About 90 percent of intestinal implants are on the colon or rectum, making something as routine as a bowel movement quite a nightmare. Symptoms can also mimic other conditions like irritable bowel syndrome, Crohn's disease, or ulcerative colitis by causing common gastrointestinal symptoms like pain, nausea, diarrhea, constipation, and even bloating. If you are unaware that endometriosis causes stomach problems it is very easy to think, "This is just my normal period," or blame it on some other stomach problem. So, yes, it's time we do talk about the poop.

Bleeding from Beyond the Vagina

Let's be serious: if you see blood coming out where it shouldn't (like your rectum), please don't shrug it off: call your doctor. Bleeding with bowel movements should never be ignored. Endometriosis can cause rectal bleeding, but so can other serious conditions like rectal or colon cancer. If this is you, don't assume it's just endo—get checked by a gastroenterologist who will likely recommend a colonoscopy to make sure we are not missing something more dangerous. Your body is trying to tell you something. Make sure you listen up.

The Bladder and All Its Parts

Like your other organs, your urinary system—is also not immune from the effects of endometriosis. The bladder (and occasionally kidneys and ureters) can host endometrial implants. Urinary endometriosis targets the bladder about 85 to 90 percent of the time, so symptoms won't stay quiet for long. When your bladder has endometriosis, it will typically send signals that can easily be confused for a run-of-the-mill UTI—this means bladder pain, frequent urination, and even blood in the urine. Painful urination that ramps up during your period is a big clue. If something feels off, listen to your bladder—it's trying to tell you something!

Infertility

Endometriosis can complicate your road to parenthood, but it certainly does not take your fertility goals out of reach. Anywhere from 25 to 50 percent of women with fertility issues have endometriosis, and 30 to 40 percent of women with endometriosis are infertile. Both mild and more severe endometriosis can interrupt the pathway to pregnancy. In mild disease, endometriosis produces toxic chemicals that impair how the ovaries function, how the fallopian tubes move, and if the uterus will implant an embryo. In later stages, the inflammation of endometriosis, large endometriomas, and thick scar tissue can distort the normal anatomy of the pelvis. This may block fallopian tubes, challenge the release of eggs, and how sperm moves through the reproductive tract. Despite all of this, with the help of a fertility specialist, many women with endometriosis are able to have successful pregnancies.

Chronic Fatigue

Chronic fatigue is a frequent companion of endometriosis. Your immune system is working overtime to manage inflammation, leaving you wiped out. This isn't just feeling "a little tired"—it's a kind of deep, bone-weary fatigue that makes doing laundry or cleaning the kitchen feel like you are scaling Mount Everest.

It can be hard to bring up feelings of exhaustion, especially when there are so many other symptoms of endometriosis that may seem more important. Do not shrug off your fatigue, it is an important part of the puzzle. You deserve to have your energy and health goals supported. Severe fatigue is a symptom that is just as important to address as your other symptoms. Don't shy away from discussing your fatigue if this is a concern for you.

Risk Factors for Endometriosis

Just like fibroids, endometriosis is a perfect storm of environment, genetics, and hormones. The biggest risk factor? Having a uterus and ovaries. The second risk factor is going through phases of your life where estrogen levels are soaring, like puberty. This is generally why we really don't see endometriosis before puberty, in postmenopausal women, or in men. What else can increase your risk? Unfortunately, there is likely no single cause.

- Endometriosis can run in the family. If your mom, sister, or grandmother have or had endo, there is a good chance you may be next in line.
- Heavy periods with bleeding lasting more than seven days.
- If your period cycle is less than twenty-seven days, you might be at higher risk.
- Starting your period before age eleven can cause a longer exposure to estrogen over your lifetime.

- A history of infertility or delayed pregnancy.
- Low body weight.
- Reproductive system abnormalities or blockages, or anything that might prevent menstrual blood from leaving your body may increase your risk of developing endometriosis.

While any of these risk factors can lay the groundwork, the true foundation for endometriosis is estrogen. Estrogen is the key hormone and when she kicks on during puberty, endometriosis can jump into full gear.

Do You Think You Have Endometriosis?

By the time many patients reach my office, they have endured a decade of pain and have seen more doctors than they can count—on average five or more—about their symptoms. Endometriosis can be a heartbreaking journey, but once it is suspected, the process for figuring out what is going on can be streamlined.

Your healthcare provider should start with a thorough medical history and exam. This means talking about your pain, period-related symptoms, and any other symptoms that might offer clues. If endometriosis seems possible it's time to initiate the "workup," or series of tests to confirm a diagnosis.

The Workup

- **Ultrasound:** This is the first-line imaging test that uses sound waves to create a picture of internal organs. An ultrasound can tell us the size, shape, and location of your uterus. It can also detail unusual findings like chocolate cysts in your ovaries. If you've got classic signs like the cysts, an ultrasound can pick them up. While ultrasounds can offer important clues, a tissue sample is still important for a diagnosis.
- **Magnetic resonance imaging (MRI):** If the ultrasound leaves questions, an MRI is the next step. An MRI uses a magnetic

field and radio waves to produce images of the inside of the body. It is an important test because the MRI image may detect concerning areas for endometriosis that are not typically seen on an ultrasound. This would be behind the uterus, the colon, and the bladder. MRIs are especially useful if we suspect advanced endometriosis or if surgery is on the table. While MRIs may be a bit more costly and/or harder to access, they are an important part of understanding what is going on inside your body prior to surgery.

- **Biopsy:** A sample of tissue from inside the body is the "gold standard" for diagnosing endometriosis. If you proceed to surgery, your gynecologist will collect several samples about the size of a sesame seed from the internal tissue to help diagnose endometriosis. After reviewing the sample under a microscope, a pathologist will confirm if it is endometriosis. These biopsies are collected either by a cystoscopy (inserting a camera into the bladder) or by a laparoscopy (a minimally invasive surgery that lets us look inside your abdomen and see the endometriosis firsthand).

- **Hysterosalpingography (HSG):** This is a test that uses special water-based dye and X-ray to evaluate the fallopian tubes and endometrial lining of the uterus. Dye is slowly injected into the uterus while an X-ray is performed to get an outline of the uterus and determine if the fallopian tubes are open. If dye is detected outside the uterus, it may mean the tubes are open for egg and sperm to meet. While an HSG cannot diagnose endometriosis, if the dye does not flow as it should, this may indicate a potential blockage or scarring of the fallopian tubes from endometriosis or other cause. An HSG is typically ordered during a fertility evaluation or if submucosal fibroids are suspected. An HSG is performed by radiologists in an outpatient setting and can be uncomfortable. Discuss ways to minimize discomfort with your radiologist before scheduling your procedure.

Take Charge of Your Pelvic Pain

For many of us, navigating the world of pelvic pain can feel like an ongoing battle. Bouncing from doctor to doctor can be frustrating and confusing as you try to understand what's going on with your pelvis. Pelvic pain is a signal your body is asking for attention. From muscles, to nerves, to pelvic organs including the uterus, ovaries, rectum, and bladder, the diagnosis of pelvic pain can be overwhelming. Despite how much effort it might take to receive a final diagnosis, your mental and physical health deserve it. Your pelvic pain is real, but so is your strength and ability to do something about it. No matter how you decide to manage and treat your condition, pelvic pain from any cause is too life consuming for you to tolerate not having a diagnosis. Advocate for yourself, trust your instincts, and do not settle for living in pain.

5

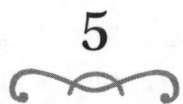

Pelvic Peaks and Valleys

Navigating the Maze of Pelvic Health

Fibroids, endometriosis, and adenomyosis are typically the usual suspects when it comes to having uterus concerns, but they are not the only issues that may have you thinking about getting a hysterectomy. In this chapter we'll shine a light on the lesser-known, but equally important conditions that could have you considering a hysterectomy: pelvic inflammatory disease (PID), pelvic floor or uterine prolapse, cancer and uterine issues during pregnancy. These are not topics that come up over brunch, but maybe they should be. We will discuss what these conditions are, their symptoms and warning signs, and racial disparities that influence diagnosis. In the case of pregnancy, we will talk about how pregnancy-related complications can impact your risk of a hysterectomy.

And yes, sometimes your conversations about hysterectomy involve the *C* word—cancer. Cancer is life changing, of course, but unfortunately hysterectomy is often a part of the treatment plan for cancers of the cervix, ovaries, fallopian tubes, and uterus. It is important that everyone with a uterus knows the warning signs and symptoms that may indicate cancer. We won't leave anything off the table even if the issues may be a little embarrassing. You need to know all your options.

Pelvic Inflammatory Disease: The Uninvited Guest

Pelvic inflammatory disease (PID), is an infection of your reproductive organs. This major pelvic infection can cause a full-blown takeover of your entire pelvis, including your uterus, fallopian tubes, and ovaries. According to the CDC, more than two and a half million women between eighteen and forty-four will deal with PID in their lifetime. In the United States this affects a staggering 4.4 percent of sexually active women and up to 10 percent women who have had an STI. Left untreated, PID is no joke.

Gynecologists are aggressive about diagnosing and treating PID, and for good reason. If left unchecked, the health consequences of PID can wreak havoc on your reproductive organs leading to infertility issues, an increased risk for ectopic pregnancy, and long-term chronic pelvic pain. PID can cause infected fluid or pus to form that spreads from the uterus to the fallopian tubes, ovaries, intestines, and rectum. This infection can turn into thin, spiderweb-like scar tissue, sticking your organs to each other. The web of scars, a classic sign of PID known as Fitz-Hugh-Curtis syndrome, can climb as high as the liver. If the infection isn't treated or is particularly bad, the thin spiderwebs become thick bands of tissue making it impossible to separate all the organs in the pelvis from one another. It is almost as if a tub of cement is poured into your body, causing your organs to stick together. We call this a "frozen pelvis," and can lead not only to chronic pelvic pain but also infertility and ectopic pregnancies.

PID is overwhelmingly caused by bacteria from sexually transmitted infections (STIs). Gonorrhea, chlamydia, or an infection known as bacterial vaginosis (BV) can work their way up into your reproductive organs and cause an infection. Occasionally, PID can occur after procedures where surgeons enter the uterus, like a D&C, pregnancy termination, or IUD insertion, and in very rare situations, bacteria from other parts of the body can cause infection.

Symptoms

Early signs of PID may be a vague, persistent abdominal pain on one or both sides of the abdomen that starts off mild and then escalates into serious pain, sometimes triggered by intercourse or even something as jarring as hitting a pothole when riding in a car. In addition to pain, PID often sends women to the ER with high fever and chills. You may have significant abdominal pain and maybe even possibly funky smelly discharge. Up to one-third of women have irregular bleeding—such as bleeding after sex, heavy or irregular periods. Others report a new sexual partner or a recent untreated infection. It is important that you do not brush off these symptoms as a simple urinary tract infection because women often have pain when they urinate or have frequent urination.

What Are the Risk Factors?

If preventing PID sounds like a good idea—and it should—then the most important step in protecting your fertility and future family planning is to prevent STIs. The major risk factors are sexually transmitted infections like gonorrhea and chlamydia, which is why we treat STIs aggressively and quickly—to prevent the development of PID.

PID is unfortunately more common in African American women and those living in the Southern United States. This is a reflection of bigger issues like healthcare access and systemic bias that delays treatment and allows progression of disease, not any genetic or biological difference. Despite overall rates of decline for PID, it remains a significant burden for women of color.

Multiple sexual partners (over a short period of time) can also increase your risk, as well as something as outdated as douching, which disrupts your vagina's natural balance. Consider this a PSA: your vagina doesn't need a car wash—it's self-cleaning. Douching, or spraying liquid into your vagina to "clean" it, disrupts the balance of vaginal flora making bacterial vaginosis more common and increases the risk for PID. Your vagina knows how to clean itself so you can leave that part alone.

A prior history of PID and intercourse without a condom are two important risk factors for PID. For this reason, your gynecologist may remind you about condom use even if they know you use another form of contraception. Condoms (outside of abstinence and mutual monogamy) are important to reduce the transmission of sexually transmitted infections. Using condoms with new partners and regularly testing for STIs so they can be treated early is important to prevent PID.

Hysterectomy in PID Treatment

Preventing PID is the most important step in protecting your fertility and future family planning, so before you panic, know that most PID cases can be treated with appropriate antibiotics and lots of patience. We understand how important your uterus is to you, however when PID refuses to cooperate and turns chronic, sometimes a hysterectomy is considered. This is the nuclear option to remove infected tissue if antibiotics aren't enough, pockets of infection called abscesses continue to increase, or if the infection spreads into your bloodstream and threatens your life. While it's not the first choice, it's on the table when health and safety are at stake.

* * *

In the end, understanding PID—and these other lesser-known conditions—equips you to tackle tough decisions head-on. You deserve straightforward answers and a say in your treatment options. Because when it comes to your pelvis, you're the host, and these uninvited guests need to know their time is up.

Pelvic Floor Prolapse: When Gravity Takes Over

Pelvic organ prolapse (POP) happens when life takes its toll on your pelvic floor muscles, and they go on strike. In POP, the once supportive "hammock-like" structures composed of muscles, nerves, and connective tissues have started to weaken, shifting your internal organs downward. Remember that your pelvic floor is responsible for keeping your uterus, rectum, bladder, and intestines in place. Weakness of the pelvic floor can make your internal organs fall (herniate), or peek out through the vagina. It is more common than you think—upward of 50 percent of women will develop POP in their lifetime, and yes, men can also experience POP. Depending on where the weakness occurs, it could be your bladder (a cystocele), rectum (a rectocele), intestines (an enterocele), or even your uterus itself can descend outside your body—this is called uterine prolapse or uterine procidentia.

Symptoms

In the early stage of prolapse, you might not even realize something is going on with your pelvic floor until your gynecologist mentions it during your yearly exam. But as the prolapse gets worse, subtlety leaves the building, and symptoms will become hard to ignore. Most commonly, you will have an unmistakable sensation that something is falling, dropping, or bulging out of your vagina. I once had a ninety-two-year-old patient describe it as "una bolita en mi vagina"—having a little ball in her vagina. This is pretty spot-on, if you ask me. It's exactly what it feels like—having a ball or bulge in your vagina pushing its way down.

This sensation is one of the most common complaints of POP. You may either see or feel tissue bulge out of the vagina. That firm "ball" could be your cervix. If you grab a mirror and look from below, you might spot a pink mass of tissue poking out, whether it's part of your bladder, uterus, cervix, or rectum. At that point, it's safe to say your pelvic floor is sending a very clear distress signal. Other symptoms include:

- **Heaviness or dragging in the pelvis:** It can feel like something is weighing down on you, pulling through your body like an anchor.
- **Bladder struggles:** Prolapse can mess with your bladder's ability to empty, leaving you running to the bathroom over and over and over—sometimes just minutes apart.

- **Leaking urine:** Laughing, sneezing, or coughing can trigger a little leak thanks to weakened pelvic floor muscles waving the white flag.
- **Constipation:** Some women even need to press on their vaginal wall with their fingers to help move rectal tissue back into place for a bowel movement—a less-than-glamorous but very real symptom.
- **Feeling as if you're sitting on a small ball:** That sensation isn't in your head—it's likely prolapsed tissue making its presence known.
- **Vaginal discomfort or irritation:** Prolapsed tissue can rub on your clothing, causing irritation or a raw feeling that is hard to ignore.
- **Lower back pain or pressure:** An unstable pelvic floor can strain your core, leading to that nagging ache in your lower back.
- **Sexual concerns:** You may feel "loose" or "open," which can understandably cause concerns about intimacy and body confidence.

If any of these symptoms sound familiar, remember you're not alone, and help is available. Pelvic organ prolapse is common, but you don't have to live with the discomfort or disruption it causes.

What Are the Risk Factors for POP?

If your pelvic floor could talk, it might say something like, "Having kids? That was a marathon, and I still need to recover." A full 75 percent of prolapse can be attributed to pregnancy and children—and the more children you have, the higher your risk. If you imagine your pelvic floor as a trampoline, pregnancy, labor, and delivery (both vaginal and C-section) are like bouncing on it nonstop. Over time the trampoline loses its bounce and will get stretched out. The connective tissue, muscle, and nerves that usually keep everything tight and lifted become compressed and can sometimes even tear.

The first bundle of joy quadruples the risk of POP and by the time baby number two comes along, your risk boosts up eightfold. Add a third or fourth child, and your pelvic floor might feel like it's auditioning for Cirque du Soleil with nine- and tenfold risk increases. Factors such as pushing for a long time (more than three hours), having a forceps delivery, a big baby, or giving birth over forty years old also increase your risk.

Now you may be thinking, "But wait, I don't have kids, so I am safe, right?" Well not so fast. Even without children, aging and menopause are enough to weaken the pelvic floor. After menopause, when estrogen levels drop, muscle can lose their strength, and for every decade you age, your risk of prolapse jumps by 40 percent. The lifetime risk of needing surgery for prolapse or related symptoms is just over 11 percent. Is this just aging or good ol' menopause? Well, the jury is still out, but either way, it is something to watch.

Our other usual suspects like chronic cough (thanks, asthma or smoking), constipation, heavy lifting, or even carrying extra weight all of which can increase your risk of POP by nearly 40 to 50 percent. If you are thinking, "My family has a history of this," you might be onto something. Some families have a history of weak connective tissue, making POP more likely. Interestingly, African American women tend to have lower rates of prolapse, while Hispanic and white women experience it more frequently. Whether it's pregnancy, aging, or genetics pulling the strings, POP is more common than we often realize—but knowledge and preventive care can go a long way.

Taking Control

Pelvic organ prolapse can be a daunting diagnosis but let me reassure you: it is not the end of the world and there are plenty of ways to manage it. If your POP is mild, intensive pelvic floor physical therapy can be a game changer. Pelvic floor physical therapy involves targeted exercises, like Kegels, to strengthen your pelvic muscles. While it sounds generally straightforward, here's the catch: Kegels must be taught and performed properly to work. It is not just about "squeeze and hope for the best."

In more moderate cases, we can recommend a nifty device called a pessary. Think of it as an elevator for your uterus. A pessary is a flat, plastic, dish-like device that sits in the vagina to keep everything in its rightful place. It's nonsurgical, easy to use, and a great solution for many women. Bonus: it can help you avoid more invasive options while still improving your quality of life.

Now, a pessary just might not cut it for the symptoms you are experiencing. If your prolapse is too extreme, surgical management including a hysterectomy may be a—dare I say—life-changing option. It frees you from the daily discomfort, worry, and inconvenience of POP—no more unexpected "drops," constant bathroom trips, or concerns about intimacy. With the right treatment, you can get back to running, jumping, and living your life without your pelvic floor calling the shots.

Get Familiar with Kegels—and Pelvic Physical Therapy

To master Kegels, a pelvic floor therapist is your best guide. First, they will help you locate your pelvic floor muscles—these are the same muscles used to stop the flow of urine. Once you have located them, the exercise itself is fairly simple: contract these muscles, hold the contraction for a few seconds, and then release. Rinse and repeat. Over time, this routine helps strengthen and tone your pelvic floor. Sometimes, your physical therapist may suggest pairing Kegels with small vaginal weights for added resistance, but you don't have to nor do you need any special equipment to get started. The best part? Kegels are quick, discreet, and can be done virtually anywhere—sitting at your desk, watching TV, or even waiting in line at the store.

But here's the thing: Kegels aren't for everyone. If your pelvic floor is too tight rather than weak, the focus shifts to relaxation. In this case, pelvic physical therapists use hands-on (and sometimes hands-in) techniques to release tight muscles and mobilize scar tissue from past injuries or surgeries. They might also introduce breathing exercises to ease pressure on the pelvic floor and evaluate your posture for imbalances that could be straining your pelvic muscles. Whether you're working to strengthen or relax, pelvic physical therapy is a personalized and effective way to give your pelvic floor the support it needs.

Cesarean and Peripartum Hysterectomy: When Plans Change

A cesarean hysterectomy, where the uterus is removed during a cesarean birth, and a peripartum hysterectomy, performed within twenty-four hours of delivery or before hospital discharge, are not what anyone imagines when drafting a birth plan, but when complications arise, surgery is typically a lifesaving procedure. Thankfully, cesarean and peripartum hysterectomies are very rare. In high-resource settings, cesarean hysterectomies occur in about 1 in 1,000 deliveries in high-resource areas, and peripartum hysterectomies are even rarer—about 0.24 to 8.7 per 1000 deliveries.

What Are the Risk Factors for Cesarean Hysterectomy?

The most common reason for both emergency procedures is the abnormal attachment of the placenta to the uterus, known as placenta accreta. This happens when the placenta embeds too deeply into the wall of the uterus and does not detach normally at the time of delivery. The placenta can embed so deeply that it grows through the uterus and into surrounding organs like the bladder. When the placenta cannot detach properly after delivery, it can cause life-threatening bleeding. In 38 percent of placenta accreta cases, removing the uterus and placenta at once is the safest course of action.

The second-most common reason is uterine atony or uncontrollable bleeding. This is a condition where the uterus doesn't close off blood vessels quickly enough after delivery of the baby and placenta resulting in excessive blood loss. This accounts for 27 percent of cesarean hysterectomies and a whopping 45.1 percent of peripartum hysterectomies. Risk factors for uterine atony include fibroids, infection, multiple pregnancies (twins or more), older maternal age, prior cesareans, and prolonged labor. While heavy bleeding can often be managed with medication or less invasive surgeries, a hysterectomy may be the only way to stop the hemorrhaging and save the mother's life.

Another significant cause is uterine rupture, where the uterus tears, typically at the site of a previous incision or C-section scar. Less commonly, cesarean hysterectomies may be required for reasons such as cervical or uterine cancer.

These hysterectomies are no walk in the park. The combination of giving birth followed by a major surgery, or having two surgeries, a C-section and a hysterectomy makes for a higher risk surgery and longer recovery. The uterus is large during pregnancy due to increased blood flow, which means a transfusion is often needed. There's also a higher chance of bladder and bowel injuries, infections, and longer hospital stays.

Cesarean hysterectomies not only cause a huge physical toll, they also take a huge emotional toll. For families that wanted more children, the sudden and permanent loss of fertility can be heartbreaking. These families often require more mental and emotional support than those with planned or elective hysterectomies. It is a life-changing event. While the hysterectomy is necessary in the moment to save a life, the aftermath can be a heavy burden to carry.

Cesarean and peripartum hysterectomies, while rare, are critical and lifesaving procedures. Understanding the conditions that may make your pregnancy high risk for a hysterectomy can help your healthcare team plan for the best possible outcomes for both you and your baby. The priority in these cases is lifesaving intervention, but taking the time to emotionally process the sudden loss of your uterus is important too. It's essential to seek support, whether through counseling or peer groups, to navigate this unexpected experience.

Gynecological Cancer

Gynecological cancer is any cancer that starts in the women's reproductive organs and includes the uterus, ovaries, cervix, or fallopian tubes. Cervical, uterine, ovarian, and fallopian tube cancers are often treated in some fashion with a hysterectomy in an effort to remove as many cancerous cells from the body as possible.

Cervical Cancer—Why Screening Matters

Cervical cancer is the fourth most common cancer in women in the world and the third most common in the United States. Despite reducing rates of cervical cancer due to screening programs, it is still the leading cause of death in forty-two resource-poor countries. Cervical cancer peaks in ages thirty-five to forty-four with the average age of diagnosis being fifty years old. The cervix is actually two parts—the ectocervix, the doughnut-shaped outer part of the cervix that can be seen during a pelvic exam, and the endocervix, a hidden canal that connects the vagina to the uterus. During your annual well woman visit, your cervix takes center stage and is the focus of the Pap smear. This simple test involves two brushes that are used to collect a sample of cells off the surface and inner canal of the cervix. These cells are only from the cervix—a Pap test is not used to detect uterine or ovarian cancer.

Here's the takeaway: a Pap smear is one of our best tools for early detection and prevention of cervical cancer. It's a simple, lifesaving test, so don't skip yours. By staying on top of screenings and follow-ups, you're taking proactive steps to keep your cervix—and your overall health—in check.

Risks for Cervical Cancer

Understanding the risk factors for cervical cancer is essential for prevention and early detection. Here's what you should know:

- **Human papillomavirus (HPV):** This is the primary risk factor for cervical cancer is the HPV virus. HPV is a common virus spread through sexual contact and directly linked to cervical, vulvar, vaginal, and anal cancer. While there are more than one hundred types of HPV, only about thirteen "high-risk" types are linked to these cancers. The HPV vaccine has been shown to protect against the most harmful strains of HPV, making this risk factor increasingly preventable. If you are eligible, please do not skip your HPV vaccination.

- **Sexual history:** Early sexual activity (before age eighteen) and having multiple sexual partners increase exposure to HPV, which increases the risk of cervical cancer.
- **Weakened immune system:** Conditions like HIV, chemotherapy, or being on immunosuppressive medication may compromise your immune system, making it harder for your body to fight off HPV infections.
- **Smoking:** Tobacco doesn't just harm your lungs—it also affects your cervix. Smoking, or exposure to secondhand smoke, increases the risk of cervical cancer by making it harder for your body to clear HPV infections.
- **Reproductive factors:** Using oral contraceptives for long periods or having many children can slightly increase your risk. The reason(s) for these associations is unclear, but it is likely the benefits of birth control outweigh this risk. You should discuss your concerns with your healthcare provider about your options and what's best for your overall health.
- **Obesity:** Obesity can complicate cervical cancer screening, making abnormalities harder to detect early. This underscores the importance of HPV vaccination, regular Pap smears, and HPV testing for all women, regardless of size.

What Happens Next?

The cells collected are evaluated to see if they are normal or abnormal. If the cells are normal then you are all set until your next scheduled routine screening. If the cells are flagged as abnormal (a condition called cervical dysplasia), you will be asked to return for a simple follow-up called a colposcopy. Don't let the name intimidate you; it's far less scary than it sounds. During this procedure, your gynecologist uses a microscope to take a closer look at your cervix and may collect a tiny biopsy (think sesame seed–size) from any suspicious areas. The results typically arrive within a week, giving you either the all-clear or a plan for further monitoring. Rest assured, cervical dysplasia does not mean cancer. It simply means your cervix is being closely watched to catch any potential issues early.

From Pap to Plan: Navigating Your Next Steps
If the colposcopy results indicate a moderate or severe cervical dysplasia, your doctor may recommend a loop electrical excision procedure (LEEP), or cold knife cone (CKC).

- **LEEP:** A thin wire loop with an electrical current is used to carefully remove abnormal tissue. It is a quick procedure done in the doctor's office under local anesthesia with minimal recovery time. If the LEEP indicates an early cancer, it is followed by a CKC.
- **CKC:** This procedure takes a more precise and deeper cone-shaped piece of the cervix to target abnormal cervical cells. Performed in an ambulatory center, it may involve slightly more blood loss than a LEEP but is equally manageable. Bonus: a CKC can sometimes both diagnose and treat early-stage cervical cancer if the entire affected area is removed during the procedure.

Symptoms
Common symptoms of cervical cancer typically include:

- **Unusual bleeding:** Bleeding between periods, after menopause, or after sexual intercourse are red flags that should be evaluated.
- **Vaginal discharge:** Increased or foul-smelling vaginal discharge that feels out of ordinary.
- **Pain:** Persistent pain in the back, legs, or pelvis that does not go away should be evaluated.
- **Systemic changes:** Unexplained weight loss, fatigue, and loss of appetite should be reported to your doctor.

- **Vaginal discomfort:** A sense of irritation or unease in the vaginal area deserves a follow-up.
- **Leg swelling:** Swelling in one or both legs is often a sign of advanced cervical cancer and should be explored.

If you're experiencing any of these symptoms, it's critical to see your healthcare provider for an evaluation. Early detection is key to successful treatment.

Hysterectomy to Treat Cervical Cancer

Here is the good news: cervical cancer can often be cured if caught early. For early stage (stage 1A to 1B2) cancer found with LEEP or CKC, surgery is the preferred method of treatment.

- **Fertility-preserving option:** For women hoping to maintain their fertility, a repeat CKC may be an option. This allows for removal of the cancerous tissue while leaving the uterus intact.
- **Hysterectomy:** For others, a hysterectomy is the preferred approach.
  - For early-stage cancer, this involves removal of the uterus and the cervix, otherwise known as a simple hysterectomy.
  - For advanced stages, a radical hysterectomy may be necessary. This more advanced procedure removes the uterus, cervix, the top one third of the vagina, and surrounding tissue.

For more advanced disease or if there is concern for metastasis, chemotherapy and radiation may be recommended after surgery. Your treatment plan will depend on the stage and extent of the disease, but early diagnosis and treatment offer an excellent chance for cure. Cervical cancer might sound scary, but with regular Pap smears and prompt follow-up, it's often preventable and highly treatable. Staying informed and proactive is your best defense.

Uterine Cancer

Uterine cancer, specifically endometrial cancer, is the first-most common gynecological cancer in developed countries worldwide, and the most common gynecological in the United States. This cancer typically introduces itself with abnormal bleeding. This can manifest as postmenopausal bleeding, bleeding between periods, or suddenly longer or heavier periods. While this cancer usually targets women between sixty and seventy years old, up to 5 percent of cases can occur before the age of forty.

Risk Factors

There has been an increase in uterine cancer over the years due to several risk factors—most involving an increase in estrogen exposure.

- **Early menstruation (before age twelve) and late menopause (after age fifty-five):** Both lead to increased exposure to estrogen over your lifetime.
- **Polycystic ovary syndrome (PCOS):** A common hormonal condition, which leads to irregular periods and higher levels of estrogen.
- **Tamoxifen:** This medication, used to treat breast cancer, acts like estrogen in the uterus and may slightly increase the risk of endometrial cancer.
- **Obesity:** Women who are obese are two to four times more likely to develop uterine cancer as fat stores increase estrogen levels in the body.
- **Family history and genetic syndromes:** Lynch syndrome and other genetic syndromes contribute to a higher lifetime risk of developing endometrial cancer.
- **Never Having Been Pregnant:** Pregnancy increases progesterone levels and gives your body a break from estrogen exposure.
- **Radiation therapy:** Radiation to the pelvis can increase the risk for cancer.

- **Medical conditions:** High blood pressure, diabetes, and gallbladder disease have been associated with increased risks of endometrial cancer.
- **Endometrial hyperplasia:** Hyperplasia is an overgrowth of cells in uterine lining and can be a precursor to cancer. If abnormal (atypical) cells are present, the risk of endometrial cancer is about 40 percent.
- **Ethnicity:** Black women are more likely to have uterine cancer than white, Asian, or Hispanic women. We are also more likely to have more aggressive cancer and higher death rates at every stage of endometrial cancer.

Hysterectomy and Uterine Cancer

The silver lining with uterine cancer? If caught early, and when diagnosed in an early stage there is a 90 percent survival rate. Treatment typically involves a total hysterectomy, often paired with removal of both ovaries and fallopian tubes (known as bilateral salpingo-oophorectomy, or BSO). In some cases, doctors may sample the lymph nodes to see if cancer has spread, meaning radiation and/or chemotherapy may be necessary. If you're premenopausal, don't worry—your doctor will work with you to discuss whether hormone replacement therapy is right for you post-surgery; if you're hoping to preserve fertility, there may be options depending on your unique situation. While uterine cancer can sound scary, the prognosis is often great, and early treatment can make all the difference.

> **Birth Control: A Secret Cancer Shield**
> *Did you know that combination birth control pills (estrogen and progesterone) can reduce your risk of endometrial and ovarian cancer? This is a little-known bonus of birth control pills. Beyond family planning, it can lower your risk of endometrial and ovarian cancer by about 50 percent. This*

protective effect lasts for ten to fifteen years even after you stop popping the pill. Talk about multitasking! So, the longer you take your trusty birth control, the more you're quietly telling endometrial and ovarian cancer: "Not today and not any day!"

Ovarian Cancer

While uterine and cervical cancers provide early clues, ovarian cancer has earned its reputation as the "silent killer" because it's often diagnosed at later stages. In the US, one in seventy-eight women will develop ovarian cancer in their lifetime, making it the deadliest gynecologic cancer.

Risk Factors

In addition to listening to your body there are several risk factors to keep on your radar:

- **Age:** If you are in your sixties or older, it's time to consider your risk. Most ovarian cancers hit after menopause, with the average age being sixty-three.
- **Family history:** If your mother, sister, aunt, or grandmother (on either side) has ovarian cancer, your risk goes up.
- **Genetic mutation:** Mutations like BRCA1, BRCA2, or Lynch syndrome increase your risk of ovarian cancer.
- **Personal history of cancer:** A personal history of breast, uterine, or colon cancer can increase your risk of ovarian cancer.
- **Ancestry:** If you are Eastern European or Ashkenazi Jewish, your risk is a bit higher.
- **Endometriosis:** Advanced endometriosis or large endometriomas have an increased risk of cancer.
- **Reproductive history:** If you have never given birth or have had trouble getting pregnant, your risk of ovarian cancer may be slighter higher.

Symptoms

You would think that ovarian cancer starts in the ovaries, but there is increasing research to suggest that some ovarian cancer might actually start in the fallopian tube. We may call this type of cancer the silent killer, but perhaps we just have to learn how to listen. While subtle, keep an eye out for these signs, many of which overlap with other cancers:

- Irregular vaginal bleeding, especially after menopause
- Abnormal vaginal discharge
- Pain or pressure in the pelvic area
- Abdominal or back pain
- Bloating
- Feeling full too quickly, or difficulty eating
- A change in your bathroom habits, i.e., more frequent or urgent need to urinate and/or constipation.

If you experience these symptoms for more than two weeks, don't just brush off what you are experiencing. Check with your doctors immediately. They will likely perform an exam and order an ultrasound, blood, and urine tests. These tests can help confirm your ovaries are normal. In ovarian cancer, early detection is key especially since there are no early screening tests, like a Pap smear.

Hysterectomy for Ovarian Cancer

Treatment for ovarian cancer almost always involves a Total Hysterectomy with bilateral salpingo-oophorectomy—removal of the uterus, both ovaries, and fallopian tubes as well as staging-removal of additional tissue and lymph nodes which might indicate the spread of the disease. And yes, chemo might follow. It's a serious fight, but with early detection, you've got a much better chance of beating ovarian cancer.

Fallopian Tube Cancer

Thankfully, fallopian tube cancer is the unicorn of gynecological cancer—it accounts for only 1 to 2 percent of all gynecologic cancers. It is often associated with ovarian cancer and therefore linked to the infamous BRCA1 gene. Fallopian tube cancer typically shows up in women between the ages of fifty and sixty, although it can occur at any age. It is more common in Caucasian women who have had few or no children.

Symptoms

Although it can mimic ovarian cancer, fallopian tube cancer has some signature telltale signs like watery or bloody vaginal discharge and swelling or a lump in the lower abdomen. Sadly, like ovarian cancer, fallopian tube cancer tends to be diagnosed late and leads to a poor outcome for most people.

Hysterectomy and Fallopian Tube Cancer

While the rarity of this cancer makes it harder to pin down exact causes and cures, the treatment approach is clear and follows the same path as ovarian cancer, including a total hysterectomy with bilateral salpingo-oophorectomy. Depending on how advanced the situation is, chemotherapy may be part of the post-surgery plan.

Vaginal Cancer

Cancer of the vagina accounts for only 1 to 2 percent of gynecological cancers, but it still packs a punch. It is less common than uterine, ovarian, and cervical cancer, but more common than vulvar cancer. While vaginal cancer is rare, it can aggressively spread to local areas including the endometrium, cervix, vulva, ovary; it can even go as far as the breasts, rectum, and kidneys.

Symptoms

Vaginal cancer can be quiet early on, but when it shows up you may notice unusual vaginal bleeding (especially after intercourse or menopause), pelvic pain, or a lump or mass in the vaginal area.

Risk Factors

Common risk factors for vaginal cancer are similar to cervical cancer as both of these cancers are HPV related:

- **Age:** It is more common in women over sixty.
- **HPV:** A history of HPV infection makes vaginal cancer more likely.
- **Smoking:** Like cervical cancer, smoking impairs your body's ability to clear HPV infections.
- **Radiation therapy:** Radiation to the pelvis can increase the risk for vaginal cancer.

Like other gynecologic cancers, early detection can improve outcomes, and because it's rare, this is a plug to keep up with your regular gynecologic exams.

Hysterectomy and Vaginal Cancer

Vaginal cancer is so rare that treatment plans depend on factors like the stage of the cancer, location, and your overall health. In the early stages, surgery is usually the go-to, with options ranging from removing just the tumor to more extensive procedures like a vaginectomy—removal of part or all of the vagina. In some cases, if the cancer has spread to the uterus, a radical hysterectomy may also be on the table.

For more advanced cases, radiation therapy in combination with chemotherapy may be used to target and destroy cancerous cells. Treatment is individualized, but the good news is that modern therapies give you options to tackle even this rare form of cancer head-on.

Vulvar Cancer

Though rare, vulvar cancer can catch women off guard, especially because it tends to show up later in life, usually after age sixty. Human papillomavirus (HPV) infection plays a major role in vulvar cancer, but it can also be associated with smoking and skin conditions like vulvar lichen scleroses. Most often, it affects the labia, but it can also make its way to the clitoris or vaginal opening.

Symptoms

Symptoms can be subtle. Look out for persistent itching, pain, or changes in the color or texture of the vulvar skin, or lumps or sores that don't heal. Any of these symptoms should bring you to the gynecologist. This is another reason why even later in life, routine visits are essential.

Hysterectomy and Vulvar Cancer

The good news is that treatment for vulvar cancer doesn't usually involve a hysterectomy. Instead, it often includes surgical removal of the affected skin on the vulva. Radiation might be necessary if the cancer is more advanced.

Empowered and Unstoppable: Your Body, Your Strength

Whether it's PID, prolapse, or cancer, the conditions that might lead to a hysterectomy aren't just medical issues—they're deeply tied to your quality of life, your self-esteem, and even your fertility. These topics can be tough to talk about, but it's critical to have all the information on the table so you can make the best decision for your health and future. And remember, there's no shame in any of this—your health comes first. The decision to have a hysterectomy may be difficult, but for many women, it can be life-changing, and in some cases, downright freeing. Whatever your journey, you deserve care, compassion, and empowerment every step of the way.

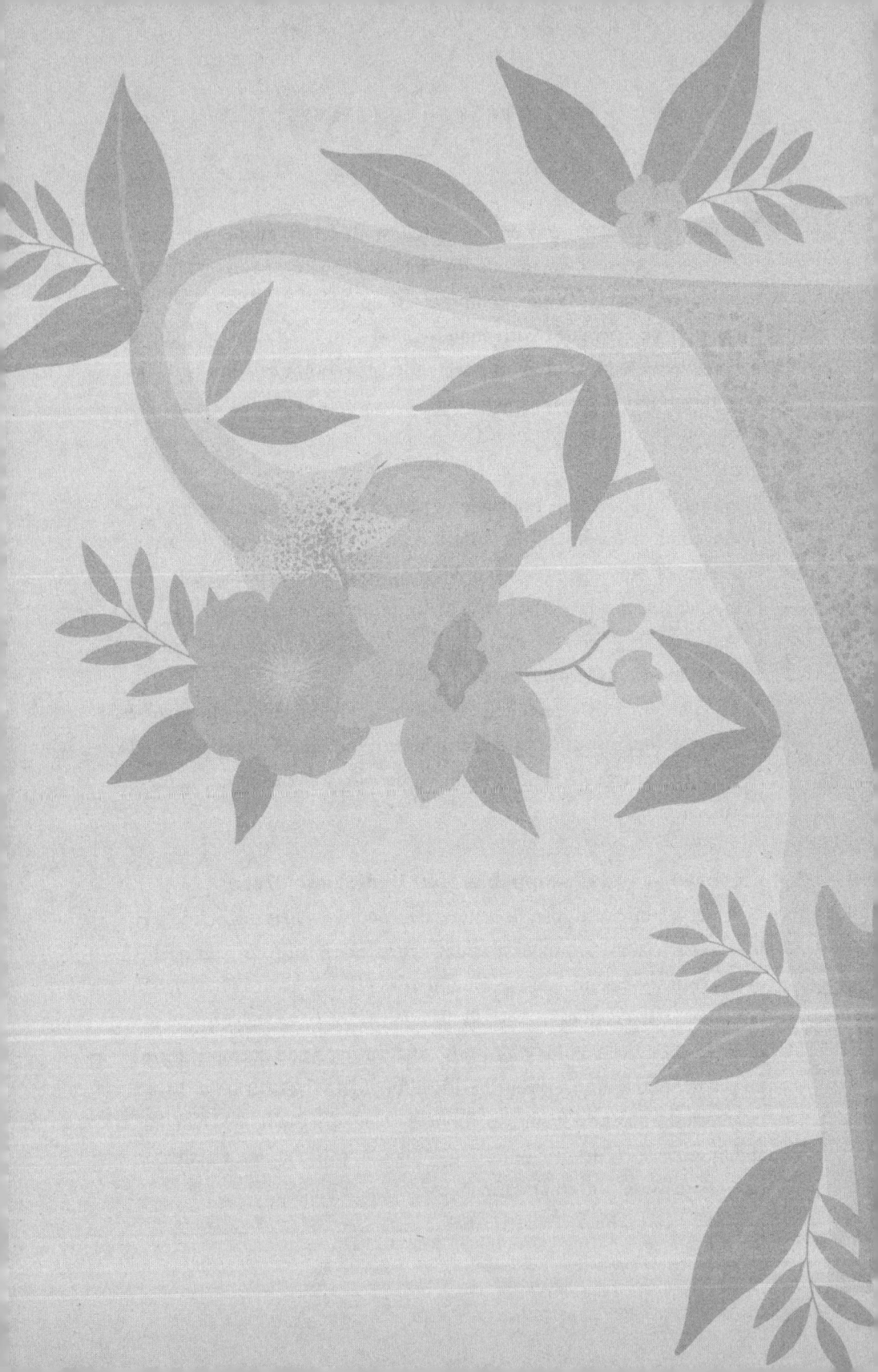

PART TWO

Your Options

6

Finding Balance

Bridging Medical Management with Holistic Options

I see patients at every stage of their health journey. Some are early in this process and simply trying to figure out why their bodies feel off. Others already know they've got fibroids or endometriosis but are intent on trying to power through life until something like the prospect of having kids forces them to confront their medical issues head-on. Then there are patients who are beyond ready for action, like a patient I saw recently who told me, "I cannot have another period, it's coming in two weeks, and I can't go through that again. I need help now."

No matter where you are on your journey, it's never too early—or too late—to learn about your treatment options. The more informed you are, the better prepared you'll be to have meaningful conversations with your healthcare team. Being proactive will empower you to advocate for yourself when you're ready to take the next steps.

While I am all about helping my patients find relief, I don't believe in fast-tracking a hysterectomy unless it is medically necessary, such as in the cases of cancer. The decision to diagnose and treat is sometimes a marathon, not a sprint. In my practice—and hopefully in the practice of medicine as a whole—we start with the simplest and least invasive solutions when we are developing your treatment plan. This often means exploring medications and lifestyle changes to address your primary concerns. Whether you prefer starting with medication, tweaking your daily habits, or are even considering minimally invasive procedures, there are many ways to tackle your medical issues without immediately jumping into major surgery.

In later chapters, we will dive deeper into minimally to moderately invasive surgical options and eventually, the "big one" itself—hysterectomy. But for now let's focus on the accessible, widely available medications and behavioral changes you can start immediately. My goal is to spark the conversation about treatment options you may have not considered or heard of before. Whether it's adjusting your lifestyle or exploring medical interventions, knowing what's on the table can be a game changer.

You are your best advocate and understanding what you can do on your own—or with the help of your doctor—will put you in the driver's seat of your health journey. Let's get started.

Medication First: Easing Symptoms, Preventing Surgery

From a medical perspective, the first line of treatment involves medication to manage your symptoms. One of the major perks? Medical treatment can keep you out of the operating room. My patients tend to love this point! As an ob-gyn, I lean heavily on medication for a few reasons, but mostly because as a guiding principle, it is smart to explore all your medical options before offering surgery. That said, there may be times when your signs and symptoms of endometriosis, prolapse, or fibroids are beyond the point where medication alone will be enough to manage them, and you may need surgical intervention first in order to improve your health.

Even in these situations, learning about your medical options is crucial. Why? Because even if you do eventually decide to have surgery, we often use medications to "keep the lid on the pot" of endometriosis flares, controlling pelvic pain, or as you plan for your surgical intervention. Surgery, whether minimally or more invasive, is a big deal. It carries risks, including adhesions (scar tissue) that can cause your organs to stick together and potentially lead to more discomfort down the road. Even uncomplicated surgeries with the best surgical outcomes can leave behind internal scars. Medications, in contrast, can sometimes treat—as in the case of endometriosis—microscopic disease we might not even see in surgery. If medication can help improve your symptoms and help you delay going under the knife, it is worth considering.

That said, medication isn't always a single, perfect solution to your complex medical needs. It can take time to find the right treatment options(s) that work best for you. There can be some trial and error. Side effects are always a possibility, which is why I've included a discussion of the potential side effects for each medication below. I also encourage you to have a healthy and open discussion with your care providers about potential side effects. Transparency builds trust and helps you know what to expect. Knowing what to expect can also make the experience of taking medication for the first time much smoother. Another downside is that some medications can only be used for a short amount of time. This can be frustrating if you find something that works wonders for you, only to have your symptoms creep back once you stop the medication.

It is also important to acknowledge the limitations of medication. While there are medications that can work wonders for heavy bleeding and chronic pain, they won't shrink a five-centimeter fibroid, move a prolapsed uterus back to place, or reverse deep anatomical changes caused by endometriosis. If you have a large fibroid pushing on your bladder or causing you to look pregnant, no medicine can remedy this—only a corrective surgical procedure will. Similarly, if your endometriosis has resulted in a large endometrioma (ovarian cyst) or deep pelvic pain, then only surgery will remove this endometrioma, reset the deep endometriosis, and restore your normal anatomy.

Using medication as a first-line treatment often also allows you to maintain your fertility. If fertility is important to you, make sure you speak to your doctor about your plans for growing your family. Medical management, however, can often suppress ovulation, making pregnancy difficult if not impossible during treatment. If fertility is a priority, it might be a good idea to engage a fertility specialist on your treatment team. After all, balancing your health issues, especially when dealing with fertility, is always a good idea.

Medication may not be perfect, but it's a valuable tool in your treatment plan. Understanding its benefits and limitations puts you in the driver's seat, empowering you to make informed decisions about your care and health goals.

But I'm Not a "Medication" Person

I meet a lot of patients who are not "medication" people. They won't pop a pill for headache, let alone for cramps or heavy bleeding. Hey, no judgment here, but let's talk real life for a second. If you had a chronic condition like hypertension or asthma, chances are you would regularly take your medication because your health—and your life—would depend on it. The same principle applies when dealing with endometriosis, fibroids, or heavy, painful periods. It's not just about managing symptoms; it's about improving your overall well-being, quality of life, and ability to fully participate in the moments that matter most.

Missing two to three days of life every month because of pain or bleeding means you are spending less quality time with your family, or at work, or even happy hour with friends (yes, that is important too!). But let's do the math: over a year, we are talking about thirty-six days of missed hugs, laughs, and sunny afternoons on a park bench. That's over a whole month of life you are giving up. You deserve better than that. You deserve to be fully present in your life, and free of the pain, bleeding, and symptoms that are holding you back.

So, if you are not a medication person I hear you loud and clear. I am not here to twist your arm. My only ask is that as you read this chapter, keep an open mind about the benefits of medicine in your life. Consider how medication might help you reclaim those lost days and avoid more invasive interventions like surgery. It's not about changing who you are—it's about opening the door to options that can give you your life back. Because you, my friend, deserve nothing less.

Pills, Patches, and Peace: Mastering Your Pain One Medication at a Time

When it comes to managing heavy bleeding or pain there are two main categories of medications: nonhormonal and hormonal. That's because your symptoms are caused first by your hormones, and then by a firestorm of inflammatory signals that light up your nerves and send SOS signals to your brain that scream, Danger, danger, you are in pain. To put out this fire, we can either tackle the hormones or cool off the inflammation—or, in many cases, do both. Hormonal medications block the whole hormonal cascade that starts the pain in the first place, and nonhormonal meds influence the pain signals in your body.

In the spirit of transparency, it is important that anytime we discuss medication you understand the potential side effects. But don't let potential side effects turn you off an entire group of medications. Remember that you are in the driver's seat. Knowing your body, medical history, and lifestyle should help you understand what might work best for you. Be open to trying something new or something you may have never heard of before, of course under the guidance of your doctor. The right treatment plan could give you back days, weeks, or even months of your life. The benefits can far outweigh the risks and this may just be the payoff you are looking for.

Taming the Flames: Using NSAIDs to Soothe Pain and Inflammation

When it comes to managing period pain or endometriosis, nonsteroidal anti-inflammatory drugs (NSAIDs) are often my go-to medications. You have probably heard of the household names for this category, including ibuprofen, naproxen, or ketorolac. These medications are like the unsung heroes of the pain-relief world, working by targeting the COX family of enzymes. COX enzymes make prostaglandins—the hormones that trigger your body's center for pain, inflammation, and even fever. NSAIDs block the COX family from functioning at full throttle and as a result they help ease pain and inflammation that come with your period.

NSAIDs don't "cure" the problem, but they can make life bearable so that you can function relatively normally. We often introduce NSAIDs at the onset of our journey because they can be very effective for controlling bleeding and pain symptoms. They are typically affordable, easy to find, and have side effects that are familiar to you—stomach upset, indigestion, and, in rare cases, ulcers. For many specialists, they are considered the first tier of medication to consider for pelvic pain, including pain caused by endometriosis.

Timing and dosing of medications is everything when it comes to taking NSAIDs. They work best when you stay two steps ahead of your pain. This means you should take them before your symptoms begin. If your cycle is regular, start a higher dose the day before you expect your period and continue taking them consistently to maintain steady levels in your system. Think of it as setting up a fortress before the pain even has a chance to attack. If your cycle is unpredictable, start NSAIDs as soon as you notice the first signs of blood or feel that familiar twinge signaling your period's arrival. Most people find they only need to take NSAIDs for the first one to three days of their cycle to keep things under control. Typically, you will only need to take NSAIDs for the first one to three days of your cycle to reach and maintain a steady level of medication in your system.

Most people tolerate NSAIDs well for short stints. Even if you are young and healthy you are less likely to have gastrointestinal side effects with short-term use. That said, there is no "best" NSAID, and some trial and error is necessary to see which one works best for you. If NSAIDs do not play nice with your stomach or you must avoid them for another medical reason, studies show that a close runner-up is acetaminophen. It does not have the same firepower of the NSAID category but is definitely better than nothing and you can avoid stomach issues altogether. All that said, NSAIDs or acetaminophen are not long-term solutions. If you find that you are taking more than the recommended amount and for a longer amount of time, it is time to go back to the medical bag of tricks and consider next steps.

Bleed Less, Live More: Antifibrinolytics to the Rescue

For many women, heavy bleeding isn't just an inconvenience, it is a full-on disruptor. Losing large amounts of blood in a short time can leave you feeling exhausted, weak, and breathless. It's the kind of issue that makes you miss work, skip social events, and struggle to keep up with family responsibilities, all while worrying about embarrassing accidents. You literally can feel like your battery has been drained. If this sounds familiar, let me introduce you to a lesser-known superhero in the work of bleeding management: antifibrinolytics.

Antifibrinolytics, particularly tranexamic acid (TXA), is a class of medication that has been quietly changing lives as far back as 1965. This hormone-free medication can work to quickly make periods shorter, lighter, and more manageable—allowing you to get back to your life and reclaim your time, energy, and confidence. For women who want to avoid hormones, daily pills, or surgery, TXA might just be the solution they've been searching for.

Here is how antifibrinolytics work: TXA helps reduce bleeding by slowing down your body's natural breakdown of blood clots. TXA blocks the breakdown of fibrin, a protein which helps strengthen blood clots. By keeping blood clots in place, the body will slow down bleeding—in this case heavy menstrual bleeding. In fact, studies show that TXA can reduce heavy menstrual bleeding by up to 49 percent and improve quality of life by 60 percent. The best part? You only take this medication while you are on your period, so there is no daily commitment. TXA is also a team player as it can be used with NSAIDs to tackle pain alongside heavy bleeding.

The advised dose is two oral pills taken three times a day for five days of menstruation. While some of my patients can feel overwhelmed by the number of pills, overall, many of them give TXA a thumbs-up for its effectiveness and convenience. If you have kidney issues your doctor will adjust the dose accordingly.

Now, let's talk about the disclosures—you know, the concerning dialogue rattled off at the end of a medication commercial while someone dances in a field of flowers. Here's the deal: Side effects are part of the package, but the goal is to keep you informed, not intimidated or scared. In research studies, the most common side effects of TXA were menstrual cramps, headache, back pain, and nausea—but these complaints were reported at similar levels in people who were not taking TXA. You should discuss with your doctor any personal history of blood clots or risk factors for blood clots like using birth control pills, obesity, and limited mobility to not further increase your risk of blood clots while using TXA. So, while it's important to know what could happen, most people find TXA manageable and effective.

Hormones to the Rescue (Just Hear Me Out)

The next line of medications is hormonal—and let's face it, hormonal treatments have gotten a pretty bad rap these days. Patients, social media, and even some healthcare professionals have declared hormones public enemy number one. I can't tell you how many times a patient has said, "I don't want to mess up my hormones," when I have offered them hormonal management for their heavy periods. Patients routinely tell me how dangerous hormones are and that they won't even consider hormonal medication. It's a common sentiment, and I get it. Hormones have become a hot topic, and skepticism is natural when you feel like they are prescribed left and right without much explanation.

And hey, I'll be the first to admit that some of my colleagues (myself included) love to prescribe hormones. I understand why this may be a source of frustration. If we aren't taking the time to explain our thought process and give you an understanding as to how and why hormones are great options, it can feel like we are not really hearing your concerns. So before you dismiss hormones outright, just hear me out for a moment.

Hormonal treatment offers a powerful, noninvasive, accessible, affordable, and most importantly, reversible option to help restore balance and control over bleeding. Unlike surgery, for the most part, hormonal treatments don't require a major commitment—they have a "fast on and fast off" effect on your body. If you ultimately decide hormones are just not for you, decide to go in another treatment direction, or decide you are ready for pregnancy, the medication can be out of your body in a matter of days.

Despite the myths and fears that continue to circulate, here's the truth: hormonal treatments have been extensively studied for decades. For otherwise healthy people, the risk of complications is relatively low.

How Hormones Help: The Basics

Let's start the discussion with the classic contraceptive pill, which has been a staple of our culture and gynecological practice since about 1960. Within two years of its introduction, 1.2 million American women were on birth control and this number has skyrocketed to more than 300 million women worldwide. The contraceptive or birth control pill is a small oral pill with a daily dose of estrogen and progestogen. Over the decades of practical use and research, the pill has become a multitasking hero in women's health. It soon became abundantly clear that there are multiple uses for the pill. The pill is not simply about preventing pregnancies, but is used to manage heavy bleeding, menstrual pain, premenstrual syndrome (PMS), and premenstrual dysphoric disorder (PMDD). The combined pill can reduce the risk of ovarian, endometrial cancers; treat cystic acne; regulate irregular periods; and more. Talk about multitasking—the oral contraceptive pill has been a game changer for millions of women worldwide.

How Does the Pill Work?

To help you understand the magic of the pill, let's think about how it interacts with the two key hormones that influence heavy bleeding and pain—estrogen and progesterone. The oral contraceptive pill delivers a steady, low dose of estrogen and progestin (a lab-made form of progesterone), which calms the brain's signals to trigger ovulation and prevent the endometrial lining from thickening excessively. The hormonal stability smooths out the dramatic hormone fluctuations that drive heavy bleeding, cramps, and inflammation.

In a nutshell, the pill doesn't just "control" your cycle—it actively lowers the overall levels of estrogen and progesterone in your system. By keeping these hormones in check, it also prevents the thick buildup of uterine lining that typically causes those extra-heavy periods. It's like hitting the "reset" button on your hormonal roller coaster, giving you a smoother, lighter, and more manageable period each month.

Reframing the Pill: Beyond Birth Control

Here is where I again ask you to think outside the birth control box—there is no one-size-fits-all for hormonal delivery systems. These methods often contain a combination of ethinyl estradiol (estrogen) and progestin (the type can vary between methods) to deliver results. The estrogen stabilizes the uterine lining, reducing irregular shedding and breakthrough bleeding. The progestin also does double duty thinning the uterine lining and prevents ovulation, making periods lighter and less painful. Together, the two work to quiet ovarian function (reduce the formation of ovarian cysts), decrease inflammation, and slow the progression of endometriosis. For many, hormonal management can make bleeding lighter, periods shorter, and sometimes even make bleeding go away entirely, depending on your unique body and needs.

Now, with that you have just learned, I hope it is clearer why "birth control" needs a new public relations team. The term "birth control" may cause a hang up about what we are attempting to achieve with this treatment. In your mind and treatment journey, moving away from this phrase is important as it strictly speaks to family planning. For you, what we are aiming to drive home is a series of steady, low-dose hormonal delivery systems that can improve your bleeding and pain experience. Instead of flooding your body with hormones—here is the twist that most of us miss—for many people the pill (and other hormonal options) lowers the amount of circulating hormones in your body. Rather than thinking we are flooding your body with hormones, we are working with your body to dial down the estrogen and progesterone levels in your body to modify your period experience.

Why Consider Hormones?
Two standout reasons make a trial of hormone delivery systems high on the list:

- **Symptom management:** These options can help with multiple symptoms at one time, including heavy bleeding, pelvic pain, and menstrual pain.
- **Customization:** There are different doses, formula options (combined—with estrogen and progestin or only progestin), and delivery systems that are available to you. If you want options, we've got options:
    - A daily combined oral pill
    - A weekly combined transdermal (skin) patch
    - A monthly combined vaginal ring

  - A quarterly progestin-only injection
  - Several hormonal progestin-only intrauterine devices or IUD

Patients often ask me, which hormonal method, specifically which pill, is best for pain, fibroids, or endometriosis. Here's the scoop: there is actually no single pill that has established itself as the best option for any one condition. Based on evidence-based research, what we aim to do is start with the lower dose of daily combined oral pill and adjust the dose of estrogen and type of progestin based on your body's response. Both continuous use of the active hormonal pill (skipping the sugar pills so you don't get a period) or cyclic use (taking the sugar pills and having a regular period) have been shown to be effective at reducing pain symptoms. Data suggests that to reduce pain and bleeding, a continuous method of use may be best.

The takeaway? Hormonal treatments like the pill, patch, ring, or even IUD are not one-size-fits-all, but they offer powerful, flexible options to help you take control of your health and reclaim your life. Whether you're managing heavy periods, cramps, or conditions like endometriosis, any of these options might just be the game changer you need.

Progestin-Only Options: A Gentle Balance

I meet patients all the time who say they have tried several pills, and nothing ever seems to work for them. Don't despair if this sounds like you. There are a variety of reasons some people cannot take or tolerate estrogen. There are still very good options to treat your bleeding or pain. We can remove estrogen from the equation and suggest progestin-only methods, such as a progestin-only pill, injection, or a hormonal intrauterine device or IUD.

Progestin is a hormone that mimics the action of progesterone, one of the main reproductive hormones made in the ovary. Progestins have been used for over fifty years to manage conditions like endometriosis and to thin the lining of the uterus which can make periods lighter and reduce bleeding. In fact, studies have shown that progestin-only treatments have similar effectiveness on pain as combined hormonal options with a bonus for improved quality of life. Some studies even suggest that progestin-only options may outperform estrogen and progestin combinations for improving pain and heavy periods. In one study, 62 percent of progestin-only users reported significant relief in pain.

Progestin-only pills are a popular once a day choice especially for women who are breastfeeding, have migraines, high blood pressure, or other medical conditions that may place them at increased risk for blood clots. If a daily pill isn't your style, Depo-Provera may be a better fit. In practice, about 50 to 75 percent of patients who use Depo for contraception have no period after four injections, or about one year of use. This makes it a great option if you do not plan on conceiving in the next few months. However, if you are hoping to get pregnant soon, Depo is a form of contraception that can linger in your body and may even delay ovulation for several months after stopping. Consider this if you are thinking about trying to conceive soon and weigh it against your other options.

As for the fine print of side effects, Depo has a notable one—irregular bleeding. This is the most common complaint and yes, it can be frustrating! It may also cause occasional acne, headaches, weight gain, and mood changes. The final notable concern is about Depo's impact on bone health. Previously the Food and Drug Administration (FDA) issued a "black box" warning about the risk of bone health, however this has since been removed. It suggested that long-term use may increase the risk of bone fractures. This limited data is countered by more robust studies noting the return of bone density after Depo is discontinued, no increased risk of bone fracture, and the support of leading organizations supporting the benefits of Depo over the risks. If Depo works well for you, it can safely be used for over two years, keeping your heavy periods in check without a daily hassle. Be sure to discuss these concerns with your doctor.

Implant and Chill: An Option to Consider

The etonogestrel implant, also known as Nexplanon or the "arm implant," is a long-acting reversible contraception that delivers a steady release of the progestin etonogestrel over the course of three years. It quietly works by suppressing ovulation, increasing the thickness of your cervical mucus, and thinning the lining of the endometrium. It is a solid choice for contraception. However, if you are aiming to manage heavy bleeding, the implant is not as powerful as the hormonal IUD or the Depo shot. Only about 22 percent of users experience no bleeding by the second year, and the chances of your period going away does not improve with continued use. That being said, about 50 percent of people do see a chance of reduction in bleeding, so it could be an option if unpredictable bleeding or spotting doesn't bother you. While it's not at the top of the list for heavy bleeding management, the implant earns a spot as a second-tier choice for symptom control. Its ease of use and long-term efficacy for contraception are definite perks, so keep it in mind if you're exploring your options!

Hormonal IUD: Set It and Forget It

As we've discussed, when it comes to managing heavy bleeding or painful periods there is no universal template for all patients to follow. Despite the availability of the combined hormonal or progestin-only options, there may be some component of trial and error until you find a treatment that is best for you. Some patients cannot tolerate estrogen, and others—like heavy smokers or those with a history of blood clots—are not suitable candidates for estrogen at all. This is where another progestin-only option comes into play: the hormonal intrauterine device or IUD. The IUD is a small T-shaped device inserted into the uterus that offers long-term, low-maintenance treatment for painful or heavy periods. For many, the IUD is the ultimate set-it-and-forget-it option to manage bleeding and pain. Despite its popularity, not everyone is an optimal candidate for an intrauterine device. Why? While the IUD can be used to treat fibroids (as well as pelvic pain, and even endometriosis), if you have fibroids your uterus may not be able to accommodate an IUD. In the best case, if you have fibroids, the height of your uterus should not be much larger than the average size of the uterus, which ranges from 6 to 9 centimeters or about 3.5 inches).

The IUD releases progestin directly into the uterus with the goal of making the endometrial lining thin and thereby dramatically controlling heavy menstrual bleeding. Depending on the IUD, you can expect a decrease in bleeding by 79 to 96 percent. In fact, one study found that by six months, over 64.3 percent of the women who were scheduled to have a hysterectomy canceled the surgery after using the hormonal IUD compared to 14.3 percent in the observation group. In larger studies, 50 percent of women had no period at all by the third month of use and 90 percent experiencing either had no period, or spotting or light bleeding only. While the IUD is not perfect—some women complain of irregular bleeding, spotting, and pelvic discomfort—many studies have shown that the hormonal IUD is a solid alternative to hysterectomy and is a very good option for controlling heavy bleeding. The IUD is an excellent option for people interested in a long-term, reversible solution that works well for bleeding and pain, without the hassle of daily pills.

Patches and Rings: Finding What Works for You

If pills, shots, and IUDs are not quite your vibe, remember that hormonal management of bleeding, fibroids, and endometriosis can come in other various forms—including patches and rings. These medications are worth keeping on your radar because of the flexibility and efficacy they offer.

Just like other hormone treatments, patches and rings use a combination of estrogen and progesterone to decrease overall hormone levels and offer flexibility to fit your lifestyle. The estrogen-progestin patch, for example, is a small medical grade sticker that adheres to your skin and changes weekly, releasing hormones directly into the bloodstream, bypassing your digestive system entirely to regulate bleeding. This is a win for those who hate daily pills or have sensitive stomachs.

The vaginal ring is a small, flexible ring, which is inserted monthly. It discreetly provides another convenient option for balancing hormones. For many, the set-it-and-forget-it convenience of a ring is a game changer. These systems not only prevent pregnancy, but they may prevent your period as well and most importantly, having options is critical. These systems offer you a range of different hormone options and delivery systems so you can find the one that best suits your body and lifestyle.

GnRH Analogues: Hormonal Healing a Different Way

For women with ongoing pain and those who have not found relief in first line treatment with NSAIDs or oral hormonal therapy—either with or without estrogen—we have to consider other strategies. Every day that passes with pain or bleeding is unacceptable. GnRH stands for "gonadotropin-releasing hormone." It is a major hormone produced in your hypothalamus. Think of your hypothalamus as the CEO of your hormonal system: it initiates the production of hormones that control hunger, temperature, fertility, and your menstrual cycle. The hypothalamus sends the GnRH signal in pulses to your pituitary gland—the middle manager of the hormonal system. The pituitary makes, stores, and produces hormones at the command of the CEO, the hypothalamus. On the command of the CEO, your middle manager, aka the pituitary gland, sends signals to your ovaries, which play the operational role in this system—to produce or not produce the hormones estrogen and progesterone.

This hormonal relay system is called the HPA or hypothalamic-pituitary-adrenal axis. In the body, GnRH medications such as leuprolide, nafarelin, and goserelin are masters of disguise and mimic the GnRH hormone. Instead of the CEO (the hypothalamus) sending pulses to middle management (the pituitary), these medications mimic GnRH and send a constant signal to change the behavior of the pituitary and ovaries. This change in signal timing (pulse versus constant) makes the pituitary and ovaries produce fewer hormones over time. For you this means less estrogen and progesterone as well as means less bleeding, pelvic pain, and symptoms of endometriosis.

When you recall what we know of fibroids and endometriosis, we learned that these conditions thrive in a higher estrogen state. Endometriosis implants not only produce, but also thrive on hormones like estrogen, sending pain and inflammation signals throughout the pelvis. In studies, we find GnRH medications are highly effective for the treatment of fibroids and pelvic pain caused by endometriosis. The primary way this is achieved is by lowering estrogen and progesterone levels to the point where these endometriosis lesions are essentially starved from the hormones that fuel them. The result includes estrogen levels that are so low that some women describe experiencing hot flashes and night sweats as if their body has entered menopause. While temporary, yes this is a common side effect. These symptoms are reversible and will improve when you discontinue using these medications.

In the US, leuprolide, nafarelin, and goserelin are all available as one- or three-month injections. These medications dramatically lower estrogen levels in the body. By drastically lowering estrogen levels, they effectively starve endometriosis of its fuel, giving you relief from pain and inflammation. Here is the twist: the estrogen levels are so low, they can cause symptoms associated with menopause. For example, up to 80 percent of women using these medications for endometriosis will experience hot flashes. Other side effects can include headache, vaginal dryness, insomnia and being increasingly emotional—all due to the low estrogen.

So, while your endometriosis may drastically improve, you may feel like you are experiencing a preview of menopause. Add to this a small chance of a degree of bone loss while you are on these medications—although it mostly improves after you stop using them. To minimize this and other bothersome symptoms risks, your doctor will offer what is called "add back" therapy. Add back therapy is when your doctor gives you a small dose of estrogen and progesterone, or progesterone only, to help protect your bones and reduce bothersome symptoms like hot flashes and night sweats. If you find these GnRH medications are working well for you, you and your doctor may decide to use them for longer with add back therapy and close attention to your bone health. Most GnRH medications are shots while the add back comes in the form of a pill. For those who prefer less juggling, newer oral medications offer a combination of GnRH analogue, estrogen, and progesterone in a daily pill. This all-in-one approach simplifies your regimen while delivering the benefits of both therapies.

GnRH medications are not one-and-done treatment options. They can also act as a bridge to fibroid or endometriosis surgery. Your surgeon may often suggest them (even for a short time) before surgery for a few reasons. When we use GnRH medications before surgery it can help shrink the size of the uterus and fibroids which can make surgery technically more straightforward and even shorter. A win-win for both you and your surgeon. It can also help stop bleeding which can boost your iron levels before surgery. Using these medications for three to six months prior to surgery can make you eligible for a minimally invasive surgery by simply decreasing the size of the uterus and fibroids. In summary, GnRH medications can help decrease your blood loss, operative time, and even rate of complication simply by making the uterus and fibroids smaller.

GnRH medications don't just stop there—they can be used for the long haul. Post-surgery, they can play offense by keeping symptoms of endometriosis that threaten to return at bay. Why? Research tells us that by two years post-surgery, more than a third of women complain of endo symptoms returning and by five years, that jumps to nearly 90 percent. For some, endometriosis just won't quit so we have to keep up the offense to protect your quality of life.

This is where GnRH medications shine. By suppressing the microscopic endometriosis left behind after surgery, your GnRH medication will help keep inflammation and pain in check, extending the peace you've earned post-surgery. So, whether you're prepping for your big surgical day or safeguarding your future from painful endometriosis symptoms, these meds should be in your toolbox. They are here to give you the best possible outcomes—before and after the OR.

Know Your Risk—Endometriosis Can Return

If you have severe or deep disease, are at a younger age at diagnosis, have had a conservative surgery (not removing the uterus and ovaries), adenomyosis, lesions on the intestines, or adhesions, hormonal suppression is definitely worth considering, even if you've had prior surgery. Hormonal suppression can be a powerful tool before and after surgery to help you fight a comeback and manage long-term symptoms.

The ultimate perk of hormonal treatments is that they offer a noninvasive way to tackle heavy bleeding and life-disrupting symptoms that come with endometriosis and fibroids. While they don't "cure" underlying conditions like fibroids or endometriosis, they can dramatically reduce symptoms including the bleeding and pain that keep you on the sidelines of life. By managing and dialing down your hormone exposure, these treatments not only relieve symptoms, but may help you steer clear of surgery, reclaim your daily life, and focus on feeling your best.

Choosing the right hormonal medication is a personal journey. The key is finding what works best for you. Whether it's a daily pill, long-term IUDs, or something in between, the right option is waiting for you. The beauty of having so many noninvasive options is that you have the power to take control of your health, reduce your symptoms, and regain your confidence in your body at your own pace. Remember, it's okay to start small. Explore your options and consider hormonal or nonhormonal treatments that align with your lifestyle before considering more drastic measures. Your body is resilient, and with the right treatment plan, you can find relief and restore balance, hopefully all without surgery.

Know that while gynecologists (myself included) may lean into hormonal management, you don't have to. You can always skip ahead to other medications or surgical management. There are times when hormones may not work, they aren't a good fit with your medical history, or you just want to proceed with surgical management first and that is okay. Hormonal treatments can be life changing in conditions like endometriosis, but that said, hormones are not a magic wand. Hormones will not improve your fertility while using them or boost your chances of pregnancy. They will not reverse scar tissue, complications of deep endometriosis, or treat endometriomas. These situations still call for surgery. Still, hormonal treatments shine as both a first step and a supporting role post-surgery, helping suppress recurring symptoms and keeping pain, bleeding, and inflammation in check. At the end of the day, the choice is yours and you must do what is right for your body. Trust your instincts and choose the path that makes you feel confident, empowered, and ready to reclaim your life.

Beyond Medication: Holistic Approaches

So many of the women who walk into my office are eager for "natural" or holistic treatments to manage heavy bleeding, fibroids, or endometriosis. Trust me, I get it. We are all eager to heal our body on our own terms. Some of this is cultural, some of this is an aversion to western medicine, and some of this might be born out of plain frustration with the medical system—the treatments you've received so far, the nonanswers you've been given. Sometimes, it's just that when our bodies turn against us, we feel compelled to find a way to fix it ourselves.

Many of us grew up on homemade remedies for everything from the common cold to a stomachache. My grandmother's remedies tasted terrible, but hey, sometimes they worked, and I felt better. These remedies were steeped in deep cultural beliefs that food and herbs are just as powerful, if not better, than the Western medicine our grandparents may not have had access to. As these tonics and tinctures were passed down through the generations, this is how we learned to treat the whole person—mind, body, and spirit. Today, as an ob-gyn, I believe in treating the whole person, not just the symptoms.

What We Mean When We Say "Holistic"

Many of us think "holistic treatment" means the traditional or culturally based herbs or practices used to treat gynecological conditions. While this can be a part of it, the definition of holistic treatment really means approaching your body and health from a lens that addresses the "whole" person. This includes your physical, mental, social, spiritual, and emotional well-being. This approach maintains that all parts of your body are interconnected, and each facet influences the other to contribute to your state of health.

Holistic treatment focuses on:

- *Lifestyle factors: This includes things like exposure to environmental toxins, diet, sleep, exercise habits, and stress levels—all of which impact your health in different ways.*
- *Alternative therapies: Incorporating techniques such as massage, cupping, acupuncture, yoga, art therapy, and music therapy can be integrated into your care plan to help support symptoms and a feeling of balance.*
- *Psychological and spiritual counseling: Holistic therapy focuses on the mind-body connection. It recognizes that your thoughts and feelings about yourself impact your physical health and encourages you to express emotions in a creative and healthy creative way.*

- *Nutritional advice: This is the emphasis on how the fuel we give our body can impact its optimal functioning. Nutrient-dense, plant-based, whole foods are crucial for the proper function of our bodies even at the cellular level.*

I fully support you taking a holistic approach to your health—just proceed with caution. Social media is overflowing with quick fix, high-cost, and too-good-to-be-true "miracle" teas and tinctures that prey on women looking for holistic answers for their health-related concerns. If something works for you and isn't causing you harm or significant expense, then proceed. If it sounds too good to be true, it probably is. Your health deserves more than a gimmick.

In my experience, the most powerful holistic approach to reproductive symptoms is making changes to your lifestyle. I believe that medication and surgery are powerful tools; however, our efforts could be for naught if we are not optimizing your diet and environment and managing your stress. Until we can identify one food, supplement, practice, or even special "diet" that can prevent or cure heavy bleeding, pain, or other gynecological symptoms—and I'm not sure we ever will—lifestyle is the best route to improving your overall health, and with it, your symptoms.

One of the most powerful holistic approaches we must employ for overall better health includes lifestyle changes that reduce inflammation. The term inflammation gets a lot of airtime these days, but let's be honest—do any of us really know what it means anymore? Let me break it down. Inflammation is your body's natural defense mechanism through your immune system. In response to an injury (cut or burn), infection (virus or bacteria), or irritation (chemical, food, or allergy) your immune system essentially sets off little fires all over the body to rally your defensive response into motion. This is great in small doses—like when you cut your finger or catch a cold. But things get messy when the fire alarm never shuts off. Over time these smaller fires never get put out and become one large, constant fire or state of inflammation. If your immune system is constantly "on," your body responds with increased levels of stress hormones like cortisol and adrenaline, which can lead to weight gain, poor sleep, heart disease and other negative changes in your heart health.

While holistic treatments cannot cure fibroids or endometriosis, taking steps to reduce inflammation through diet and lifestyle can make a really positive impact on these conditions. To live an anti-inflammatory lifestyle you should routinely ask yourself, "Does [insert food, drink, activity, thought, medication, et cetera] contribute to an anti-inflammatory lifestyle?" Will it improve how your body functions? Will it decrease stress and improve your well-being? Will it help you sleep? These are all questions you can ask yourself as you redesign your life to help you fight damaging inflammation.

Four Factors for an Anti-inflammatory Lifestyle

1. Nutrition

After caring for so many women dealing with fibroids, endometriosis, and pelvic pain one thing is crystal clear—so much healing starts in the kitchen. Maintaining an anti-inflammatory diet is important for your reproductive and general health now more than ever before. Many of us grew up with little to no say about what we ate or how it was sourced. If your upbringing was anything like mine, you probably did not learn much about nutrition and the importance of the fuel we put into our bodies. You may have not learned about "clean eating," organic produce, veganism, or any other variation of a healthy diet until you were in college or even in older adulthood. Let's face it, now most of us are playing catchup after years of eating the standard American diet or what is mockingly called the SAD diet—a diet high in processed foods, fast foods, animal protein, sugar, saturated fat, and sodium. Conveniently named, right? But it's never too late to pivot and optimize the power of nutrition so you can take control of your symptoms and find relief.

Your diet is the first place to start. I am going to sound like a broken record but: plants, plants, plants! This is the first place to start when trying to level up your anti-inflammatory lifestyle. Plant-based, plant-forward, or vegetarian—whatever you want to call it, eating more plants is where it's at. The research is unanimous—a plant-based diet works to decrease the buildup of inflammation in our bodies. Plants are rich in antioxidants, which are fancy nutrients that pick up "free radicals" or chemicals that damage your cells and DNA. We need an abundance of antioxidants to counteract the stress signals that impact the way our cells function and DNA replicates. If these stress signals are left unchecked, they can lead to disease and cancer.

You see, certain proteins like the COX-2 family and prostaglandins—yes, the same ones tied to painful periods—are also tied to inflammation. Plants reduce inflammation by decreasing prostaglandins, nitric oxide, and COX-2 proteins. Plant-derived proteins can suppress the production of these pain signals and as a result decrease inflammation all over the body.

We also know that your digestive system isn't just about breaking down food. There is an exciting body of evidence showing that the bacteria in your intestines—also known as your gut flora—have a massive impact on your immune system and how your body responds to stress. A plant-forward diet, which is naturally high in fiber, helps your gut produce flora that counteracts inflammation in the body. This not only has the potential to help you manage your inflammatory symptoms like pain but also strengthens your immune system, making your body more resilient against chronic diseases like obesity, heart disease, dementia, and even fibroids.

As for red meat, the verdict is still out. What we do know from studies is that women who consume meat have a higher incidence of fibroids and other negative health-related conditions. There is an increased risk of chronic diseases like type 2 diabetes, cardiovascular disease, and colorectal cancer in processed and unprocessed red meat eaters. It will not be a surprise if endometriosis and fibroids are added to this list in the upcoming years.

So, what is the goal here? To increase the number and variety of plants that you eat every week to, in turn, decrease inflammation in your body. I tell all my patients to "Eat the rainbow" and more specifically, aim to eat at least thirty plants—both fruits and vegetables—a week with a focus on the most colorful (hence the rainbow), nutrient-dense, and low-sugar options. That's right, not all fruits and vegetables are created equal. For instance, purple and red berries, and yellow and orange fruits and vegetables contain both natural antioxidants as well as polyphenols—all of which are great for fighting inflammation. Dark green leafy vegetables are rich in vitamin K, antioxidants, and iron. Studies have noted that an increase in cruciferous vegetables like broccoli, kale, cauliflower, cabbages, and fruit like apples and tomatoes may lower the risk of developing fibroids. While the exact mechanism needs to be explored, it is suggested that it's possibly because these fruits and vegetables not only help detoxify the body, they also remove excess estrogen from your system. It doesn't end there. Pears and apples contain a flavonoid called phloretin. Phloretin contains anti-inflammatory properties that help prevent chronic disease and it also serves as an estrogen blocker—a hormone we know influences fibroids.

Sipping on green tea may also be your new weapon for fibroid health. Green tea is not only one of the most popular drinks in the world, it is loaded with numerous antioxidants that may counteract estrogen's effect. When it comes to antioxidant fighting power, green tea even outshines vitamin C. The primary antioxidant in green tea is epigallocatechin gallate (EGCG), a powerhouse antioxidant that has shown potential in animal studies by blocking pathways that lead to tumor growth. Intrigued? So are we.

In a small, but fascinating randomized controlled trial, thirty-nine women with fibroids were split into two groups: one that received a daily supplement of 800 mg of EGCG daily for four months, while the other did not. The results are encouraging. In the untreated group, 24.3

percent saw their fibroids grow, while 32.6 percent of women in the EGCG group experienced a decrease in fibroid size. Even with this small size of this study, the difference is statistically significant. Even more promising is that the women taking EGCG reported a significant improvement in their symptom severity and quality of life.

While it's important to note that this was a small study—meaning more research is needed before we can call green tea a miracle cure—it's an exciting glimpse into how plant-based nutrition may help reduce inflammation and promote health. So, the next time you have the urge to drink a soda versus brewing a cup of green tea, sip with purpose— your body just might thank you.

When it comes to revolutionizing your diet to combat inflammation there is still more you can do. Think of whole grains as your foundation. Whole grains and starch options like brown rice, quinoa, and barley aren't just tasty; they're packed with nutrients and fiber to support a healthy gut and keep inflammation down. For an added boost, toss in some flaxseed. Not only are they an excellent source of fiber, but research suggests they may even inhibit estrogen sensitivity in the uterus—a win for anyone looking to minimize the impact of their food on the body.

Also remember to spice things up. Spices like turmeric and ginger are well-known anti-inflammatory heavyweights and can easily be incorporated into our daily meals. While you are reanalyzing what is in your refrigerator, let's not forget about your gut. The gut is quickly emerging as the unsung hero of your immune system and should be a huge target of anti-inflammatory efforts. Fermented foods like yogurt, kefir, sauerkraut, and kimchi are teeming with "good" bacteria. These probiotics work like an army, supporting gut health and helping your body fight inflammation from the inside out. As you reconsider the concept of inflammation, think of your diet as part of your tool kit—you are equipping your body with everything it needs to combat daily inflammation. And while it may seem like new territory, experimenting with grains, seeds, spices, and fermented foods is a good place.

Vitamin D often comes up when we talk about hormones. And while there is no such thing as a "hormone balance," I often find that patients are frankly vitamin D deficient and these deficiencies do play a role in health optimization, especially when it comes to fibroid management. Vitamin D has shown promise in protection against chronic conditions. Here's a key point to consider—people with richly melanated skin often have lower levels of vitamin D because their skin is less efficient at producing it from sunlight. This puts them at a higher risk of deficiency compared to their lighter-skinned counterparts.

Several studies have suggested a connection between vitamin D deficiency and an increased risk of fibroids. While we're still waiting on larger-scale studies to confirm the extent of this link, there's no harm in being proactive. Boosting your vitamin D levels can be as simple as soaking up a little sunshine, incorporating vitamin D–rich foods into your diet (hello, cashews and hazelnuts!), or adding a supplement to your routine. Talk to your doctor before you start a supplement, but typically 600 IU daily is recommended. Think of it as a low-risk, high-reward strategy in your fibroid management plan. So if a handful of nuts, a daily vitamin, or a walk in the sun can help you potentially avoid invasive treatments, isn't it worth a shot?

What About Soy and Dairy?

Soy is also having a moment in health circles and research groups and for good reason. Whether in the form of tofu, soy milk, edamame, tempeh, and miso, soy is one of the most popular, plant-based sources of protein. If you don't think soy is in your diet, think again—you are more connected to soy than you think. While 6 percent of the world's soybeans are directly consumed by humans, the rest sneaks into the food chain in our beef, chicken, eggs, and dairy, vegetable oil, margarine, chocolate, ice cream, baked goods, cosmetics, and soaps; the list goes on and on. So yes, we all probably consume more soy than we think.

Soy is popular for being a versatile and nutrient-dense phytoestrogen. Phytoestrogens (plant-based compounds that mimic estrogen in the body), are subjects of growing research as this may be helpful to some postmenopausal women, but not so much for women in their reproductive years dealing with estrogen-sensitive conditions such as endometriosis or fibroids. Isoflavones—a subset of phytoestrogens—like genistein and daidzein found in soy may function like estrogen in the body and have a complicated role in fibroid growth. There is data to suggest that genistein can affect fibroids once they are formed, but the particular dose that influences this effect remains unknown. Daidzein is another well-known isoflavone of interest found in soybeans. Its by-product, equol, is made in the intestines and has an even stronger estrogen activity than daidzein. In some aspects it may even be considered an endocrine disruptor due to its ability to interact with estrogen receptors all over the body. While equol may be helpful in some health settings like menopause, there is a potential risk for women of reproductive age with fibroids. All this early emerging research needs to be further explored in larger studies, making this ever more complicated. To date, there is no single food or compound alone that causes either endometriosis or fibroids.

When we consider the intersection of your diet, the gut microbiome, ethnicity, genetics, age, and the environment, understanding these conditions becomes much more complicated. So, is soy safe? The jury is still out. If you enjoy soy-based foods and they fit into your lifestyle, there is probably no need to totally abandon them, but like with most things in life: moderation is key.

Dairy is another category where moderation is important. Dairy products are staples in many diets, but they're notably hormone-rich. The relationship between dairy and fibroid *health isn't entirely clear-cut, but it is worth paying attention to how dairy affects your body so you can make adjustments to improve your health. Organic, grass-fed, or hormone-free dairy may offer a healthier alternative for you if you aren't ready to give up dairy altogether. Interestingly, data from the Nurses' Health Study suggests a protective effect of dairy, primarily from yogurt and perhaps more specifically calcium, which interacts with how your body processes vitamin D, and may help reduce the risk of developing fibroids. In a different population, the Black Women's Health Study suggests that any dairy intake, regardless of fat content, was associated with fewer fibroids. In the US, where Black women typically have lower intake of dairy than white women, understanding the role of dairy in the development of fibroids is critical.*

2. Move Your Body

Movement and exercise are powerful tools for fighting inflammation. Aerobic exercise in particular—anything that gets your heart rate up—helps fight chronic inflammation by reducing body fat, which activates anti-inflammatory pathways in your body and increases hormones and chemicals that reduce inflammation. Exercise also helps manage pain, especially during your menses.

Regular exercise—at least forty-five to sixty minutes of aerobic activity three times a week—is nonnegotiable. The beauty of exercise is that you have options. Vigorous cardiovascular exercise like running, cycling, or high-intensity interval training (HIIT) workouts are particularly useful for weight loss and increasing your body's anti-inflammatory hormones. They're also known to boost endorphins, which act as natural pain relievers during your period. If you are not a fan of boot camp, or it is not appropriate for your level of fitness, then lower intensity exercises like brisk walks, yoga, and swimming are also a good way to reduce stress, support anti-inflammatory hormones in the body, and help with pain from cramping. Figure out what is best for you—consistency is key so make it something you know you can stick to.

3. Sleep Hygiene Is Everything

Many—if not most of us—do not get enough sleep on a daily basis. I can relate to the frustration of endless nights lying awake in bed. We mentally plan the day to come and review our lengthy to-do list, battling the anxiety that comes along with it. When sleep finally comes it is just a matter of time before a hot flash, a partner's snoring, or a child climbing into our bed interrupts our sleep. Falling back to sleep again? Basically impossible. Sleep deprivation can take a toll on your body and to many it is unknowingly a form of stress.

Long-term lack of sleep harms the body by chronically raising your cortisol levels. Cortisol, a stress hormone, can actually make us more resilient in short, intermittent bursts, like the kind you get from exercise, but when consistently high it can weaken your immune system, increase inflammation in your body, and even cause high blood pressure. Sleep deprivation can also stimulate stress and anxiety in chronic pain, endometriosis, and fibroid patients which may exacerbate symptoms. Sleep deprivation can worsen pain sensitivity, too, which creates a vicious cycle of pain and worsening symptoms.

Maintaining consistent and restorative sleep is essential for controlling symptoms and enhancing overall quality of life when you're dealing with endometriosis and fibroids. It's just as important to your health as regular exercise. Your body needs anywhere from seven to nine hours a night in a cool, dark, quiet room with the same sleep and wake up time every day for optimal functioning. Some tips for maximizing your sleep include:

- Avoid naps lasting two or more hours especially during the daytime.

- Go to bed and wake up at the same time each day even on the weekends.
- Avoid strenuous exercise within one hour of going to bed.
- Avoid staying in bed longer than you should two or three times a week.
- Steer clear of anything that may alert or stress you before bedtime.
- Avoid going to bed feeling stressed, angry, upset, or nervous.
- Reserve your bed for sex and sleep only.
- Maintain a comfortable bed and bedroom environment (temperature, light, noise).
- Avoid important work before bedtime and avoid working in bed.
- Avoid thinking, planning, or worrying when in bed.

Implementing these habits can help you achieve the restorative sleep you need to manage both pain and stress.

4. Embrace Mind-Body Practices

Chronic stress, which is common when you've spent years struggling with pain and heavy bleeding, is pro-inflammatory. It can make your symptoms worse, and it's also linked to other inflammatory conditions like depression, inflammatory bowel disease, cardiovascular disease, and rheumatoid arthritis. It's worth it to seek out opportunities to manage your stress, and with it your inflammation. Mind-body practices like meditation and mindfulness have been shown to promote relaxation and studies even show fewer inflammatory markers in those who participate in them. They help you feel safe and grounded in your body, manage busy, anxious minds, and connect you with the creative, confident, resilient, and joyful parts of yourself.

These practices fall under a wide umbrella—everything from acupuncture to yoga and from mindfulness practices to tai chi have been shown to help us manage stress, reduce inflammation, and minimize pelvic pain. They include relaxation, hypnosis, visual imagery, meditation, biofeedback, cognitive behavioral therapies, group support, and spirituality as well as art therapy like art, music, or dance. Even simple breathing exercises you can do at home will help you reduce your stress.

What to Avoid

I've been giving you helpful tools to incorporate into your life to fight inflammation, but now it's time for tough love. There are some behaviors that we should all ditch—if you haven't already, like yesterday.

Processed Foods

Let's start with processed carbohydrates—such as potatoes, bread, and rice are nothing but empty calories that spike your blood sugar and provide minimal to no nutritional value. Fried and processed foods—think anything that comes out of a package or a box—nope, they don't love you either. Red or processed meat? Same story. And finally, processed sugar and alcohol—okay, you get my point, but I'm shouting this from the rooftops for the folks in the back: these foods don't do you any favors when it comes to improving your health or well-being.

But let's also be real about something else—it's hard to avoid these foods. For so many reasons it is really hard, if not impossible, to avoid some of these foods. Culturally, rice and bread are intertwined in most of our meals, celebrations, and are staples in meals across the globe. Red meat is a centerpiece of many diets, especially in the US. Then there's the emotional side. On a day when life feels like it's giving you a one-two punch, there's a certain kind of magic in fast food, a heaping plate of white rice, or—for me—a salty bag of chips. These foods bring comfort when we need a quick pacifier for stress, and that's okay sometimes.

Let's get something straight: making the switch from a processed-food diet to a cleaner, healthier one is no walk in the park. This isn't about pretending it's easy or expecting a miraculous overnight transformation. It's about taking small, intentional steps that focus on progress, not perfection.

Start by targeting the biggest troublemakers: sugary drinks, packaged snacks, and fast food. These guys are villains of the world of inflammation. Replace them with simple, doable swaps. Water instead of soda. Fresh fruit instead of candy bars. Whole foods you genuinely like instead of something that comes vacuum-sealed in plastic. Your taste buds will adapt, and soon enough, these changes will feel like second nature.

Now, let's talk about dairy. This all depends on how it makes you feel? If you're bloated or sluggish after indulging in whole fat dairy or processed cheese, consider cutting back—especially on nonorganic options. That creamy latte or double helping of cheese? It might need to step aside for your anti-inflammation goals. The key is to experiment and listen to your body. You don't have to say goodbye to every indulgence forever, but you'll find that even small adjustments can make a big difference. Every choice you make is a step toward feeling better, and that's a journey worth taking.

Smoking

Sis, are you still smoking? Oh honey, it is time to let that go. Cigarette smoking or vaping is a big no-no if you are trying to optimize your health. We have known for decades that the toxins in tobacco smoke cause cancer and that nicotine is seriously addictive. That is not breaking news, but here is the plot twist: not only is nicotine addictive, it is actually toxic to the immune system. Nicotine and the other toxins in cigarette smoke convince your cells to make and send out inflammatory markers like it is their full-time job. In addition to triggering your immune system, research has shown that the heavy metals in cigarette smoke may impact reproductive conditions. For example, increased levels of the metal cadmium in the blood is associated with a significantly increased risk of endometriosis. If you are serious about an anti-inflammatory life, it is time to kick your cigarettes and vape pen to the curb.

Targeted Nutrition for Endometriosis

Women with endometriosis are often misdiagnosed with a myriad of gastrointestinal issues for years before the correct diagnosis is made. Over the years many women have learned to turn to nutrition-based approaches to complement medical treatments. Two common dietary approaches include the endometriosis diet and the FODMAP diet, both of which offer relief but in different ways.

The FODMAP diet targets digestive issues that may overlap with conditions like IBS. This diet restricts certain types of carbohydrates that are difficult for some people to digest. These carbohydrates are called FODMAPs (fermentable oligosaccharides, disaccharides, monosaccharides, and polyols) and are short-chain carbohydrates (sugars) that can lead to bloating, gas, and stomach pain.

Here's a more accurate breakdown, starting with foods to limit or avoid if following a low-FODMAP diet.

- **Dairy (high in lactose):**
  - *Milk*
  - *Yogurt*
  - *Ice cream*
- **Wheat products (high in fructans):**
  - *Bread (especially white or whole wheat)*
  - *Cereal*
  - *Crackers*
- **Beans and lentils:**
  - *Legumes like chickpeas, kidney beans, and lentils (high in GOS—galacto-oligosaccharides)*
- **Vegetables:**
  - *Artichokes*
  - *Asparagus*

- *Onions*
- *Cauliflower*
- *Garlic*
- **Fruits:**
  - *Apples*
  - *Cherries*
  - *Pears*
  - *Peaches*
- **Foods with high-fructose corn syrup:**
  - *Sodas and processed foods*

And here are some low-FODMAP foods, which are (safer options for those following the diet):

- **Dairy (lactose-free or low-lactose):**
  - *Lactose-free milk*
  - *Lactose-free yogurt*
  - *Hard cheeses like cheddar or parmesan*
- **Wheat-free or Low-FODMAP grains:**
  - *Gluten-free bread*
  - *Corn flakes, oats, and quinoa*
  - *Sourdough spelt bread (low in fructans)*
- **Beans and lentils (in small amounts, if tolerated):**
  - *Canned lentils (small amounts rinsed thoroughly)*
  - *Firm tofu and tempeh (low in FODMAPs)*
- **Vegetables:**
  - *Carrots*
  - *Zucchini*
  - *Spinach*
  - *Bell peppers*
  - *Cucumbers*

- **Fruits:**
  - *Bananas (unripe)*
  - *Blueberries*
  - *Strawberries*
  - *Pineapple*
- **Sweeteners:**
  - *Maple syrup*
  - *Rice malt syrup*
  - *Table sugar*
  - *Dark chocolate (in small quantities)*
- **Nuts and Seeds:**
  - *Macadamia nuts*
  - *Peanuts*
  - *Pumpkin seeds*
  - *Walnuts*

After eliminating certain foods, they are slowly reintroduced. If any reintroductions cause abdominal pain, they are forever eliminated from the diet.

The endometriosis diet is not as rigid a diet but is consistent with the anti-inflammatory theme we have been focusing on; it emphasizes anti-inflammatory, fiber-rich food with restrictions on processed and red meats, dairy, gluten, trans fats, and refined sugars. In essence, the endometriosis diet is essentially a blend of anti-inflammatory, hormone-supporting, and gut-friendly foods that aim to reduce the inflammatory load on the body. It can be challenging to judge the overall effectiveness of the endometriosis diet as the diet can vary from person to person. However, in limited studies patients have reported an improved quality of life when following this approach.

Both the endometriosis and FODMAP diets have their strengths and choosing the best one often depends on the primary symptoms you're experiencing. If inflammation and hormonal concerns are at the root of your pain, the endometriosis diet may offer more targeted relief. If digestive pain and bloating are your main challenges, then perhaps the FODMAP diet can provide relief, especially if gut issues make your endometriosis symptoms worse.

Because both diets involve significant food restrictions, working with a registered dietitian to ensure you're meeting your nutritional needs while addressing your reproductive health needs is recommended. Whether you choose one diet, or a mix of the two, the goal is the same: to reduce pain, promote healing, and improve your quality of life.

* * *

I invite you to listen to your body. As you navigate the path toward managing your health, remember that you hold the power to choose what you put into your body to optimize your health. Hormonal treatments can offer relief, but they are just one part of the equation. Holistic approaches, from nutrition and movement to mindfulness, are powerful tools that can help you to take control of your health in ways that align with your beliefs and lifestyle.

As you consider hormonal medication or experimentation with lifestyle and dietary changes, or a combination of the two, be sure to engage your healthcare professionals so you stay healthy and safe. Each journey with fibroids, pelvic pain, or endometriosis is unique and that is okay. Figuring out what works for you and finding success with medication, lifestyle change, or a bit of both will go a long way in helping you understand your body, what it needs, and how to optimize your reproductive health.

7

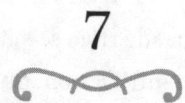

What to Consider First

Minimally to Moderately Invasive

I recently had the pleasure of operating on one of my most lively patients, a critical care nurse named Chelsea who is no stranger to medicine, the operating room, and post-op care. The week before the surgery, she came to the office for her preoperative visit and we shared a hearty belly laugh about what she affectionately called her "fibroid babies." She was beaming as she talked about finally evicting the fibroids that have been a drag on her life for years. Chelsea was emotionally exhausted from fielding questions from her coworkers, like "Are you pregnant?" and fed up with random strangers asking, "When is the baby due?" For years, her fibroids had caused chronic constipation and exhaustion, heavy monthly bleeding that made her exhausted, and impacted her high-stress job. Chelsea was ready to reclaim her life—one fibroid-free day at a time.

Despite recommendations from several other medical professionals that she undergo a hysterectomy, we went in a different direction: an abdominal myomectomy, a collective decision that was aligned with her values and desire to maintain her fertility. "Look," she said, "I haven't thrown in the towel yet. My eggs aren't all scrambled, and I still want to make some babies." An abdominal myomectomy is a procedure that kicks fibroids to the curb while leaving your uterus intact, keeping the door open to explore motherhood later on if desired. As a savvy health professional, Chelsea was familiar with a hysterectomy. She had hoped to avoid it for herself but had already tried several medications that failed to help results symptoms to her satisfaction. She put up a fight against the heavy bleeding, but ultimately after we were unable to stop her relentless symptoms, we knew it was time to move on to more aggressive treatment. She needed something in between medication and hysterectomy.

Maybe you are Chelsea or can relate to her story. Have you seen several doctors who have tossed around the word *hysterectomy* a bit too casually? In the back of your mind, you probably know that surgery is likely in your future, but you just aren't ready to take the leap. You have to embrace your own journey, and I understand that. Maybe you have tried multiple medications and dabbled with holistic treatments, and only recently have started to entertain the idea that something more definitive may be on the horizon. If this sounds familiar, this chapter is for you. Here is where I hold your hand as we move beyond medical treatments and lifestyle changes and explore all the options from the least to most invasive on the surgical spectrum. You deserve to know what's available before going all in on a hysterectomy, and I am here to make sure that you do.

In the world of medical procedures, we can think of your options along a continuum. On one end, there are less invasive treatments with no abdominal incisions to deal with; these treatments involve techniques that use special imaging, heating techniques, or even treatments performed through the vagina. Then we have the other end, with more invasive procedures involving tiny incisions on your body (sometimes with the assistance of robots—because we do live in the future). Then at the far end of the spectrum, there are procedures that require we use larger incisions. It may seem overwhelming, but trust we are going to break it down and keep things simple. In the following pages, I will guide you through all the available options so you can make the best choice that aligns with your values, your body, and your future.

As we dive into these more invasive options, it is ever so important to find a care provider who can dance—and yes, I mean dance—with you. This is a collaborative practice we call shared decision-making. While it can take time, it is totally worth the effort to help you arrive at a health-care treatment plan that you are comfortable and on board with. Here is how the dance of shared decision works. As your doctor I suggest a treatment that can help treat the symptoms that are most bothersome to you. From here you step in to share the thoughts, feelings, and values that make you interested (or not) in this treatment plan. We talk through the pros and cons of the plan, you ask questions and consider how it respects your health goals and lifestyle. We may go through a few rounds of this before we find our rhythm, but in the end, you are not only well informed about your options, but you are making a decision that feels right for you.

This is shared decision-making in a nutshell—a back-and-forth dance that you and your physician do until we get into rhythm of collaboration, mutual respect, and progress toward your health goals. Chelsea and I did this dance for a few months (per her own timeline) until she came to the decision to move forward with an abdominal myomectomy. Trust me, with time and the right healthcare team, you will find your own groove.

Many of the minimally invasive options we will explore are focused on managing bleeding and fibroids. Endometriosis, on the other hand, is a slightly different beast. With the management of endometriosis, we often lean on medication to treat pain, bleeding, and pelvic pain symptoms. If this fails, surgery—including resection of endometriosis and the option of a hysterectomy—can be considered as a last resort. We start with minimally invasive treatments either over your abdomen or through a vaginal approach that can treat bleeding, pain, and fibroids.

Informed Consent

Before diving into any gynecological procedure, it's essential to fully understand the full picture—this includes the risks, benefits, and alternatives to the procedure. This is what we call informed consent and it plays a crucial role in helping you make decisions about your health. Whether you're considering a minimally invasive option or a more extensive option, it's important to have a clear understanding of what exactly each procedure involves. How will the procedure affect your symptoms? What is recovery like? What are the possible complications? Will this procedure impact my fertility? These questions, and so many more, are key to knowing if the choice you are making is right for you. Informed consent is when you and your doctor get into the nitty-gritty detail of the surgical process. Your doctor will guide you through the pros, cons, and alternatives of medical treatments or the surgical process. You can then make a well-informed decision to move forward or even decline treatment. This discussion may require more than one office visit. Why? You will likely have questions, and we want to give you space to process our dialogue and manage expectations about surgery and recovery. As you decide what treatment is right for you, the informed consent process ensures you are an informed patient and that your concerns about your body and surgery are addressed upfront.

Your Options, in Brief

In the following sections, we'll explore each of these procedures in detail. For now, here's a quick guide to get you started.

- **Magnetic resonance–guided focused ultrasound (MRgFUS) or high-intensity focused ultrasound (HIFU):** Outpatient procedure with focused high-intensity ultrasound waves used over the abdomen to heat and destroy fibroid tissue.

- *Procedure time:* 1.4 to 4 hours
- *Hospital days:* 0
- *Return to normal activities:* 1 day
- *Advantages:* Same-day procedure requiring no hospitalization, no incisions, no radiation, and no general anesthesia. Low complication profile and quick return to daily activities from the next day of treatment. May help avoid a more invasive procedure.
- *Disadvantages/risks:* Size and location of fibroids impacts if they can be treated. Fibroids may recur with time. It is a safe procedure with minimal risk; however, infrequent complications are abdominal pain/cramping, back or leg pain, urinary tract infection, vaginal discharge, skin injury (burns), and transient nerve damage.
- *Future fertility:* Unpredictable effect on fertility.

- **Uterine artery embolization (UAE):** An outpatient procedure that involves using small particles to block the blood vessels that supply the uterus. This may not only cause fibroids to shrink in size but also result in less menstrual bleeding overall.
  - *Procedure time:* 30 minutes to 1.5 hours
  - *Hospital days:* 0 to 1 day
  - *Return to normal activities:* 3 to 10 days
  - *Advantages:* No abdominal surgery needed and a relatively quick recovery. May avoid a more invasive procedure.
  - *Disadvantages/risks:* Low risk of inducing menopause if beads travel to and block ovarian blood supply. Possible surgical risks include bleeding, infection, blood clots. Bleeding may return over time.
  - *Future fertility:* Unpredictable effect on fertility.

- **Hysteroscopy D&C:** An outpatient, minimally invasive procedure that involves looking inside the cavity of the uterus and sampling the lining of the uterus with a spoon-shaped instrument.

- *Procedure time:* 15 to 45 minutes
- *Hospital days:* 0
- *Return to normal activities:* 1 to 2 days
- *Advantages:* Allows us to directly look into the uterus to ensure tissue that needs to be removed is not missed and that a comprehensive sampling of the uterine cavity is completed. May avoid a more invasive procedure.
- *Disadvantages/risks:* Risk of injury to the uterus, infection, and risk of anesthesia—all of which are low.
- *Future fertility:* If too aggressive, a D&C can damage the lining of the uterus and impact future fertility.

• **Operative hysteroscopy:** Similar to the hysteroscopy D&C, an operative hysteroscopy allows for the removal/resection of a polyps and fibroids under the direct visualization of the instruments.
  - *Procedure time:* 15 to 45 minutes depending on the size of the polyp/fibroid and the fluid restrictions of resection system that is used.
  - *Hospital days:* 0
  - *Return to normal activities:* 1 to 2 days
  - *Advantages:* Operative hysteroscopy allows for direct removal of polyps or fibroids without disturbing the rest of the cavity if desired. May help avoid a more invasive procedure.
  - *Disadvantages/risks:* Risk of injury to the uterus, infection, and risk of anesthesia—all of which are low
  - *Future fertility:* If too aggressive, a resection may damage the lining of the uterus and impact future fertility.

• **Endometrial ablation:** An outpatient, minimally invasive procedure that uses water, vapor, or other medium to destroy the lining of the uterus (endometrium) to reduce or stop heavy menstrual bleeding.

- *Procedure time*: 15 to 45 minutes or less, depending on the method used.
- *Hospital days:* 0
- *Return to normal activities:* 1 to 2 days
- *Advantages:* A minimally invasive procedure that may decrease vaginal bleeding. May help patient avoid a more invasive procedure.
- *Disadvantages/risks:* Risk of injury to the uterus, infection, and risk of anesthesia—all of which are low. Not suitable if you wish to become pregnant as pregnancy afterward is not recommended. Bleeding may return and other intervention is required.
- *Future fertility:* Pregnancy is not recommended after this procedure and effective contraception is recommended.

- **Radio frequency ablation (RFA):** A minimally invasive procedure using heat generated by radio waves to destroy targeted tissues, often used for fibroids or bleeding management.
  - *Procedure time:* Approximately 30 to 60 minutes
  - *Hospital days:* 0
  - *Return to normal activities:* 1 to 2 days
  - *Advantages:* This procedure is minimally invasive with quick recovery. It may effectively reduce bulk symptoms and pain. May help patient avoid a more invasive procedure. The procedure can be done under local or general anesthesia.
  - *Disadvantages/risks:* May require laparoscopic surgery. Potential for infection, bleeding, or burns to surrounding tissues. May not work with large fibroids, multiple fibroids, or fully eliminate symptoms, requiring further treatment. Should complete childbearing before considering this treatment.
  - *Future fertility:* Fertility is not guaranteed or encouraged after RFA; pregnancy is possible but may be high-risk.

- **Myomectomy:** Surgical removal of fibroids from within the uterus. Several surgical approaches: open/abdominal, laparoscopic, and robotic.
  - *Procedure time:* 1 to 3 or more hours
  - *Hospital days:* 0 to 3 days
  - *Return to normal activities:* 2 to 6 weeks depending on approach used
  - *Advantages:* This is a day procedure requiring possible hospitalization. Depending on the procedure type may remove all fibroids and improve anatomy.
  - *Disadvantages/risks:* Fibroids can regrow, and/or all fibroids may not be removed resulting in recurrent symptoms and additional procedures. Pain of recovery, risk of infection and anesthesia. Possible surgical risks include bleeding, adhesions, and infections.
  - *Future fertility:* Possibility of pregnancy after adequate healing time. A cesarean section may be required for delivery.

- **Hysterectomy:** Removal of the uterus with or without the cervix. There are several surgical approaches, such as vaginal, abdominal, laparoscopic, and robotic.
  - *Procedure time:* 1.5 to 3 hours
  - *Hospital days:* 1 to 3 days
  - *Return to normal activities:* 2 to 6 weeks depending on approach used
  - *Advantages:* This is considered definitive treatment as the uterus is removed. The ovaries may be removed or spared.
  - *Disadvantages/risks:* Reproductive potential is lost. Side effects may include early menopause and a reduction in libido—if ovaries are removed. Possible surgical risks include bleeding, infections, adhesions, injury to the intestines, or bladder.
  - *Future fertility:* Reproductive potential is lost.

High-Intensity Focused Ultrasound (HIFU) or Magnetic Resonance–Guided Focused Ultrasound (MRgFUS)

When it comes to cutting-edge fibroids treatments, high-intensity focused ultrasound (HIFU) and magnetic resonance–guided focused ultrasound (MRgFUS) are both high-tech cousins of traditional imaging studies performed by a radiologist. They harness energy-based methods without the need for a knife. Intrigued? Let's get into these treatments:

High-intensity focused ultrasound (HIFU) is a noninvasive treatment primarily developed and used in China.

- *The setup:* For this procedure you lie on your back while an ultrasound probe directs high-frequency ultrasound waves aimed directly through the skin and to the fibroids.
- *How it works:* High-frequency ultrasound waves are aimed directly at fibroids. The ultrasound energy generates heat which targets and destroys the fibroids.
- *The catch:* While promising, HIFU is mostly limited to China and hasn't gone global. That means data and access are still limited, making it more of a "good to know" option than a mainstream choice.

Magnetic resonance–guided focused ultrasound (MRgFUS) is perhaps the shiny, newer extension of HIFU. MRgFUS takes HIFU a bit further and pairs two radiologic technologies: ultrasound and MRI.

- *The setup:* For MRgFUS you also lie on your back but inside of an MRI machine which will locate your fibroids.
- *How it works:* Over the course of a two-to-three-hour treatment, the built-in ultrasound probe uses real time thermal monitoring from the MRI to precisely target and destroy individual fibroids.
- *The catch:* Although FDA approved access is limited in the United States and most insurances still consider this technique experimental.

Who's a Good Candidate?

These futurist treatments may not be for everyone, but they can shine for people who have access and other favorable traits. Here is what early data suggests are the best candidates for this high-tech solution:

- **Size matters:** Smaller fibroids respond better to treatment, as they're easier to target and shrink effectively.
- **Location is key:** Fibroids closer to the abdominal surface are easier to target with ultrasound waves versus fibroids in the back of the uterus or near a sensitive structure such as the bladder.
- **Blood supply:** Highly vascular fibroids (rich in blood flow) are prime candidates since these treatments rely on heat delivery via blood flow to destroy fibroid tissue.
- **Adenomyosis:** If you have this condition alongside fibroids, you're more likely to experience significant relief from pain and heavy bleeding.

So, if your imaging (MRI or ultrasound) matches these criteria, MRgFUS could be a game changer for managing your symptoms. As for HIFU, it's worth keeping on your radar—especially if you're traveling to places where it's more commonly available.

Pros and Cons

Both HIFU and MRgFUS are exciting high-tech options, but are they really worth it? Let's break down the pros, cons, and practicalities of either procedure so you can decide if either of these is right for you.

HIFU: Low-Risk, but Limited Access

Why it's appealing:

- HIFU has an exceptionally low risk of complications, making it a safe option.

- Most patients experience minor side effects, such as skin burns, changes in menstrual bleeding, or mild discomfort for a few days.
- HIFU may avoid the need for more invasive surgery.

The downsides:

- Access is the biggest hurdle. HIFU is primarily performed in China, making it a challenge for most patients outside the region. This also limits the data we have on the success, best candidate, and long-term outcomes of the procedure.
- Costs are hard to estimate but likely high for those traveling internationally for treatment.

MRgFUS: Low-Risk, Big Cost

Why it's appealing:

- FDA-approved for fibroids that can be accessed by ultrasound
- MRgFUS may avoid the need for surgery.
- Clinical studies report that 70 to 80 percent of women experience improved symptoms and quality of life.
- Targets fibroids individually, minimizing risks to nearby organs like the ovaries, reducing the chance of ovarian failure.

The downsides:

- MRgFUS works best on smaller fibroids because the treatment time for larger fibroids would be longer than three hours.
- MRgFUS works best with fibroids near the abdominal surface. Deeply embedded fibroids or ones near critical structures like the bladder, colon, or nerves may not be treatable.
- Treatment of large fibroids may be partial, leading to size and symptom reduction but not full resolution of symptoms.

- Costs range from $15,000 to $25,000 and are rarely covered by insurance due to its experimental status and extreme cost.
- While the procedure is effective for many, 20 to 30 percent of patients may require additional treatment within three to five years, adding to the financial burden.
- Specialized radiology training is required.

The Recovery

HIFU is an outpatient procedure that uses limited sedation, no skin incisions, does not require a hospital stay, and has a generally quick recovery. You should plan to be back on your feet in a matter of a few days with minimal discomfort.

MRgFUS is also an outpatient procedure requiring one to two days of recovery. However, everyone is different and total recovery time could be, on average, about 1 to 2 weeks.

Bottom Line

If you're hoping to avoid surgery and have the means to access these options, MRgFUS could be a game-changer, especially for smaller, accessible fibroids. But with limited access, high costs, and insurance challenges, it's worth considering more established procedures that may be covered, even partially, by insurance. These treatments are exciting advancements, but they come with significant hurdles—both logistical and financial.

Uterine Artery Embolization (UAE)

This is a popular, outpatient intervention (sometimes advertised as a uterine fibroid embolization, or UFE) performed by radiologists. A UAE works by blocking major blood vessels that bring blood from the body to the uterus. By significantly decreasing the blood flow to the uterus, fibroids no longer have the fuel to grow. After this procedure—theoretically—the ultimate goal is stunting the growth of fibroids and relief from heavy menstrual periods.

- *The setup:* For this procedure you should start with a consultation with your gynecologist to discuss your short- and long-term fertility plans. If you are no longer childbearing or have no plans for children, then an interventional radiologist will order an MRI to assess the size and location of your fibroids. If you are having heavy bleeding along with your fibroids it will be important to make sure there is no underlying endometrial cancer (this can be done with a simple office procedure—a pipelle biopsy) before proceeding with the UAE.
- *How it works:* After informed consent, you will be brought into the operating room where you will lie on a specialized table. First up, your anesthesiologist will give you either local or general anesthesia to make sure you have a pain-free experience before the procedure starts. Once you are relaxed and comfortable, the radiologist will step in. The radiologist will make a small incision near your groin where they will access the superhighway of blood vessels that lead to the uterine artery. Using a specialized X-ray machine (a fluoroscopy machine, if we are being technical) your doctor will take several images to map out the path to your uterine arteries on both sides of your body.

  Once the arteries are located, the radiologist will inject small plastic or gelatin-like particles. These particles will stick to the vessel wall and will eventually form a roadblock to blood flowing through the artery on the right and left side of your body. The fluoroscopy machine helps confirm that there is no blood flow. After both sides are blocked, the catheter is removed, and light pressure is held on your groin for about five minutes. The procedure takes about sixty to ninety minutes. After you have recovered from anesthesia, you will be discharged to your home with pain medications and strict instructions to relax and recover.

- *The catch:* While uterine artery embolization (UAE) has earned its spot as a popular fibroid-busting procedure, let's set the record straight: it's best reserved for women who have finished their childbearing journey.

Here's the deal: Radiologists are rock stars at what they do, but fertility and reproductive health? That's your gynecologist's stage. The lens through which a radiologist views UAE is purely technical, while your gynecologist sees it through the prism of your long-term fertility and pregnancy goals. And trust me, those lenses aren't interchangeable.

Why does this matter? Let's talk about the rare but real risk: in some cases, those tiny UAE beads meant to block blood flow to fibroids can wander off to the ovarian artery. The result? Unplanned menopause and irreversible fertility loss.

I've seen too many young women go through this heartbreak after choosing UAE without consulting their gynecologist first. Don't let that be your story. Before committing to any procedure, bring your gynecologist into the conversation. They'll help ensure the treatment aligns with your future plans—whether that's baby-making, symptom relief, or both.

Bottom line? UAE is a fantastic option in the right circumstances, but your gynecologist is your ultimate fertility bodyguard. Don't skip that crucial chat!

Who's a Good Candidate?

Uterine artery embolization or UAE, is a minimally invasive treatment for heavy menstrual bleeding and (depending on the location) for those vexing "bulk" symptoms associated with fibroids—like pelvic pressure, urinary frequency, and even the belly pudge that makes people (rudely) say, "Hey, I didn't know you are pregnant!"

This procedure may be your uterus saving MVP if you:

- Have heavy, long, or painful periods from fibroids or adenomyosis—enough already, right?
- Have "bulk" symptoms—we are talking pelvic pain or pressure, enlarged belly, incontinence, or constipation. Ugh, thank you fibroids.
- Have completed or do not desire childbearing
- Are pre- or perimenopausal and want to keep your uterus. It's been through enough already.
- Are not the best candidate for surgery—for example, anesthesia is risky for you, you have uncontrolled hypertension or diabetes, or you just want a less invasive option.
- You want or need to minimize your time off from work, because life doesn't stop for fibroids.
- Have several smaller to moderate-size fibroids versus one giant, troublemaker fibroid.
- Have a uterus below the belly button.

If any of this sounds like you, consider a Uterine Artery Embolization as an option to slow the tide of blood and shrink those fibroids—all while avoiding surgery and keeping your uterus with you!

Pros and Cons

Uterine Artery Embolization is popular in my practice, but like anything it may or may not be the best fit for you. Whether you are a good candidate will depend on the size and location of your fibroids, how heavy your bleeding is, as well as how significant your bulk symptoms may be to determine whether this is the best procedure for you. Here are the up and downsides that you need to consider before making any major decisions.

Why UAE is appealing:

- **High success rate for bleeding relief:**
  - Most patients will have some improvement after a UAE. As early as the first year after treatment, upward of 90 percent of women see a reduction in bleeding—this is an immediate and gratifying win for you.
  - 73 to 90 percent of women report improvement or resolution of heavy bleeding, with results lasting up to 10 years in some cases. Depending on your age and results, this is a long amount of time to have an improvement in your symptoms and most importantly avoid surgery.
  - Improvement for some women was so significant that they canceled plans for a hysterectomy.
- **Improvements in bulk symptoms:**
  - 89 to 91 percent of women notice relief from pressure and urinary issues.
  - Ultrasounds confirm fibroid shrinkage in most cases, especially for smaller fibroids.
  - Large fibroids may not see as significant a reduction in size.
- **Minimally invasive:**
  - This is a minimally invasive procedure with no incision on your abdomen—only a small incision near the groin.
  - There is a short recovery time compared to hysterectomy or myomectomy.
  - Most procedures are outpatient or require just a twenty-four-hour hospital stay.
- **Less blood loss:**
  - Reduced bleeding compared to abdominal surgeries.
  - Helpful for women needing preoperative preparation before a larger surgery. If you currently have anemia, a UAE can slow monthly menstrual bleeding to help resolve your anemia and prepare you for a larger surgery if desired.

- **Presurgery perks:**
  - Uterine artery embolization can sometimes be used before major abdominal procedures like a myomectomy, hysterectomy, or even cesarean section.
  - Prior to a bigger, more invasive surgery a UAE can help decrease blood loss during the larger surgery. A UAE can also help decrease the size of the uterus. Moving from a large, bulky uterus to a smaller uterus may make the more invasive surgery safer and more manageable.
  - Can improve the chances of laparoscopic surgery (by reducing the size of the uterus) instead of an open procedure.
- **Cost and accessibility:**
  - Often covered by insurance, making it a budget-friendly option for fibroid management.

The downsides:

- **Post-embolization syndrome (PES):** About one-third of patients experience PES making it the most common post-procedure downside of UAE. PES is the onset of moderate to severe cramping, pain, severe nausea, vomiting, or loss of appetite as the uterus tissue is deprived of blood and may start a few hours to days after the procedure. Just under 10 percent of patients need to be admitted to the hospital for a day or two for IV pain or nausea medication to manage these symptoms until they pass.
- **Infection:** There is a small risk (0.9 to 2.5 percent) of infection.
- **Loss of fibroids:** Depending on the size and location of the fibroids, small pieces of fibroid may be expelled or released through the vagina. This occasionally may require another surgery (a dilation and curettage) if they do not come out on their own or completely.

- **Damage to nearby structures:** While rare, there is a small risk of injury to surrounding structures, especially blood vessels.
- **Need for repeat treatment:** If symptoms do not improve, you may choose to go back for a repeat procedure or proceed with another option altogether.
- **Risk of premature menopause:** This is a big one, especially if you want to have a baby in the near or distant future. There is a 7 percent risk of ovarian failure in women over the age of forty-five. While we do not have reliable statistics in younger women, it is estimated that the risk of premature menopause is 1 to 3 percent. Young women are more likely to recover from ovarian injury than younger women, but it is not guaranteed.
- **Pregnancy risks:** While data is conflicting, there is evidence that after a UAE, you may have an increased likelihood of miscarriage, preterm delivery, low birth weight of your baby, C-section, and postpartum hemorrhage. This is why it is important to make sure that you consult with your ob-gyn prior to this procedure and have completed your childbearing before proceeding with a UAE.
- **Fibroid Size and location are key:** Similar to other procedures, patients have better outcomes with small to moderate-size fibroids. Large fibroids may not shrink sufficiently to alleviate your bulk symptoms entirely.

Recovery

After the procedure, you'll head to the post-op recovery area for a few hours to shake off the anesthesia. Think of this as your "Netflix and chill" time—but without the Netflix and with one rule—to keep your legs straight. We want to give your groin incision the priority treatment while it heals from the procedure.

Depending on your center, you may stay overnight for some extra TLC (and pain management), or you might be sent home with a prescription for oral nausea and pain meds—remember one third of patients may experience the post-embolization syndrome and need fast treatment.

Once you're home, and comfortably situated in the bed or on your couch, light tasks like answering emails or organizing your snack stash are fair game. By day eight, you should be feeling more like yourself, and most women are back to work within ten to fourteen days—just in time to remind everyone how fabulous you are and (hopefully) heavy bleeding and painful period-free!

Dilation and Curettage (D&C) and Hysteroscopy

Dilation and curettage—commonly known as a D&C, "scraping," or biopsy—is a well-established procedure that gynecologists use to help diagnose and treat heavy bleeding by removing endometrial tissue from inside the uterus.

- *The setup:* An appealing aspect of a D&C is that it is generally a quick and straightforward procedure. Gynecologists can perform the procedure in or out of the office to gather very helpful information about your bleeding and to even treat your bleeding.

  This procedure is crucial in evaluating heavy or abnormal bleeding because a significant sample of endometrial tissue can be sent to the lab for analysis. The goal is to ensure there are no pre-cancerous or cancerous conditions causing your bleeding. A D&C also allows your gynecologist to remove irregular menstrual tissue or polyps that can cause your heavy or irregular bleeding.

- *How it works:* A dilation and curettage is a two-part procedure; dilation involves gently opening the cervix to allow for instruments to pass into the uterus, while curettage is when a rigid, spoon shaped instrument known as a curette passes into the uterus to remove endometrial tissue.

  Sometimes, you will hear the term hysteroscopy attached to dilation and curettage. After dilating the cervix, we can then pass a hysteroscope—a thin, lighted camera—through the cervix and into the uterus. We fill the uterus with saline and inflate the cavity like a balloon which allows us to scope out any polyps or fibroids that require special attention to remove.

The image inside your uterus is projected real time onto a screen where we can see the entire uterus and even the opening of your fallopian tubes. This live feed allows us to precisely guide our instruments to remove polyps or fibroids, ensuring we remove tissue from every part of the uterus with special attention to problem areas. After looking, the camera is removed and the curettage or scraping completes the sample of the endometrial lining.

- *The catch:* Fortunately, dilation and curettage is a very straight forward procedure. There aren't many "gotchas" here to catch you up. Occasionally, a condition called cervical stenosis can happen—this is where the "doors" of the cervix are sealed preventing the passage of our surgical instruments. This can happen without a reason, in women with prior cervical surgery, or postmenopausal women. Occasionally, your doctor may prescribe medication called misoprostol to help soften up the cervix to allow for safe passage through these "doors" and into the uterus.

Who's a Good Candidate?

If you are thinking about a hysteroscopy dilation and curettage, it's important to make sure you're a good candidate. Here are a few scenarios to consider:

- There is suspicion of a fibroid or polyp that needs to be removed.
- We need to confirm your bleeding is not due to cancer.
- You have anxiety or concerns about having a biopsy in the doctor's office and would like anesthesia for the procedure.
- An attempt at an office biopsy was unsuccessful either because you were uncomfortable, the cervix would not open (cervical

stenosis), or there was no tissue removed during the biopsy attempt.

- You have a normal-size uterus to adequately visualize the inside cavity.

Pros and Cons

A D&C can be a quick solution to stop heavy, ongoing bleeding especially if bleeding has not responded to other medical treatment. For some, it may be a great bridge to temporarily manage bleeding as you and your doctor develop a more long-term plan—especially if you are showing signs of anemia (weakness, fatigue) from the loss of blood. Your gynecologist might even suggest placing a hormonal IUD after your procedure to keep the lining of the endometrium thin with the goal of reducing ongoing heavy bleeding.

Why it's appealing:

- **Quick and simple:** Hysteroscopy and dilation and curettage are fast, straightforward procedures typically performed in an outpatient setting. It does not typically require a heavy lift from patients in terms of time off work.
- **Comfortable with anesthesia:** Intravenous or general anesthesia ensures comfort and reduces the chance of movement, helping protect the uterus from damage during the procedure.
- **Effective for heavy bleeding:**
    - Can quickly stop bleeding, especially in cases of anemia-related fatigue or weakness.
    - Often used as a bridge to help manage symptoms until a more permanent solution is implemented.
- **Low infection risk:** Performed in a sterile operating room, with such a low risk of infection that antibiotics are generally unnecessary.
- **Immediate relief with long-term options:** Reduces heavy bleeding quickly, with the option to place a hormonal IUD during the procedure to help keep the uterine lining thin and prevent future bleeding.

- **Diagnostic and therapeutic:** Allows for tissue sampling to rule out conditions like endometrial cancer or to remove fibroids or polyps.
- **Minimal recovery time:** Recovery is typically mild, with patients waking up comfortable and ready to return to your normal light activities within a day or two.

The downsides:

Many patients don't find a big downside to a D&C unless there is a complication, or your bleeding continues and you're forced to move to a more invasive procedure(s).

- **Not a permanent solution:** While it can alleviate symptoms, a D&C may not always address the underlying causes of heavy bleeding, such as fibroids or hormonal imbalances.
- **Risk of uterine damage:** Rare but possible risks include perforation or damage to the uterine lining during the procedure. You will be consented for this before you start the procedure.
- **Anesthesia risks:** As with any procedure involving anesthesia, there's a small chance of complications like reactions to medications.
- **Temporary discomfort:** Mild cramping or light spotting may occur post-procedure, though usually manageable with over-the-counter pain relievers and resolved by the time you leave the out-patient center.
- **May require further treatment:** For some, additional procedures may be needed if symptoms persist or if the underlying condition isn't fully resolved. This may be a reason to insert a hormonal IUD: to discourage the return of more bleeding and extend the positive improvement of bleeding most experience after a D&C.
- **Limited Scope:** Best suited for smaller uterine abnormalities; larger or deeply embedded fibroids may require a different approach.

Recovery

After any hysteroscopy (with or without D&C), you may experience some very mild cramping—nothing an over-the-counter medication like ibuprofen can't handle. Most of the time, patients wake up very comfortable. There's an extremely small risk of infection but make sure to give your doctor a ring if you have any abdominal pain, fever, chills, or foul-smelling discharge in the days and weeks following your procedure.

A little light bleeding may be expected for about a week or so after the D&C. This is totally normal. As a general rule of thumb, if you are bleeding enough to fill two regular-sized pads over one hour or two hours, or if you feel lightheaded, dizzy, or faint, then call your doctor, stat. These are signs that your bleeding is more than what we would typically expect from this procedure.

Most importantly, do not forget your follow-up appointment. One of the main reasons for the procedure is to figure out why you are bleeding, whether it's polyps, fibroids, precancerous or cancerous tissue. Your tissue results, also known as the pathology results, are typically ready seven to ten business days after the D&C, if not sooner. The results help determine the next steps of treatment so keep in touch with your doctor to make sure your results are benign and also to keep your bleeding in check.

Operative Hysteroscopy

Not only can we look inside your uterus with a small camera, but we can also remove fibroids and polyps from the uterus at the same time. This technique is called an operative hysteroscopy and is a game changer for bleeding.

- *The setup:* The procedure provides an opportunity to control bleeding by removing fibroids and polyps in the lining of the uterus through a minimally invasive vaginal approach.
- *How it works:* Similar to a hysteroscopy, we insert a camera into the uterus which is inflated with saline (clear solution of water and salt) so we can clearly see inside the uterine cavity. With the uterus

distended we have a crystal-clear view of everything inside that can cause bleeding. The best part is that once we identify what needs to be removed, a special handheld device is inserted through a small channel in the hysteroscopy camera to remove or resect a fibroid or polyp right on the spot. These handheld devices typically involve an electrical, self-contained cutting system that shaves down fibroids and polyps until the area is flush or smooth with the normal uterine wall. The smaller fragments are then suctioned out of the uterus. This handheld device may also be referred to as a resectoscope. A resectoscope is an electric wire loop that "resects," or cuts, the fibroid in pieces that are then removed. In many ways, it is an extension of an operative hysteroscopy, and the end goal is the same. If a fibroid is removed, this procedure is called a hysteroscopic myomectomy, and if a polyp is removed, it's called a hysteroscopic polypectomy.

Who's a Good Candidate?

We communicate about the location of fibroids based on the International Federation of Gynecology and Obstetrics (FIGO) classification system. Using this classification we are able to understand the fibroid location that is most amenable for removal by hysteroscopy. The most favorable fibroids for resection are those closest to or inside the uterine cavity, otherwise known as FIGO type 0, type 1, or type 2. Don't worry too much about the categories; it really just comes down to how much fibroid is in the cavity that we can access to remove. To know if you are a good candidate for this relatively safe, fast, and effective procedure we have to determine the size and location of your fibroids. There are a few ways we can do this: a transvaginal ultrasound, MRI or even an in-office SIS (saline infusion sonohysterography or saline infusion sonogram).

Pros and Cons

If more than half of the fibroid is inside the muscle of the uterus (not hanging out in the cavity), I inform patients that we may not be able to resect or remove the entire fibroid at one time. This is because it is simply not safe to burrow too deep into the muscular wall of the uterus to remove the entire fibroid. If this is the case, symptoms may still occur, and we might have to return for another resection as the uterus pushes more of the fibroid into the cavity for us to access. Size is an important factor here as well. There is a risk of incomplete removal in fibroids larger than 2 inches or about 5 centimeters so understanding where and how large your fibroids are prior to this procedure is important in anticipating outcomes.

See below figure for a visual:

Type	Description
0	Pedunculated intracavitary
1	Submucosal <50% intramural
2	Submucosal ≥50% intramural
3	Contacts endometrium 100% intramural
4	Intramural
5	Subserosal ≥50% intramural
6	Subserosal <50% intramural
7	Subserosal pedunculated

Just like the other procedures we have discussed, anesthesia is needed. In the office setting, it can be as straightforward as numbing medication on the cervix and intravenous (IV) sedation. In an outpatient surgical center, you'll receive general anesthesia. There are a few techniques used to perform an operative hysteroscopy, so it is important to discuss with your doctor what is the best option for you, especially if you have plans for fertility in your future.

Recovery

After this procedure, many patients see an improvement in their bleeding profile pretty quickly. A hysteroscopic myomectomy or polypectomy is also safe for future pregnancy and comes with very little risk of infection or uterine rupture—a complication we will talk more about when we discuss abdominal myomectomy.

Saline Infusion Sonohysterography or Saline Infusion Sonogram (SIS)

An SIS is a procedure that helps diagnose conditions in the endometrium or lining of the uterus. During an SIS, sterile saline is slowly injected into the uterine cavity with a thin catheter. As the cavity expands, we can use the ultrasound machine to check for any irregularities—like polyps or fibroids—in the endometrial lining. SIS is a quick and easy way to figure out what is going on in the lining to help us plan which surgical approach is best for you.

Endometrial Ablation

An operative hysteroscopy or hysteroscopic myomectomy is not the only minimally invasive vaginal option available to you. Another alternative is an endometrial ablation. This is a promising option to tackle bleeding, polyps, and fibroids. The endometrial lining has two parts: a superficial (top) functional layer which produces menstrual tissue and supports pregnancy, and a deeper basal (basalis) layer, which regenerates the top functional layer after your period or a pregnancy.

- *The setup:* The goal of ablation is to selectively damage both layers and stop regrowth which—theoretically—should lead to lighter or perhaps no period at all. Of course, before we offer an ablation, we have to make sure you are not bleeding from a precancerous or cancerous condition. This requires a small biopsy of the endometrium before the ablation because if there is cancer then an ablation is off the table. If your biopsy is normal, you are in the clear and can proceed with an ablation. There are several ways to perform an ablation: with radiofrequency energy, heat, and cold. All have the same goal: to destroy the endometrial layers that support the production of your menses. Be sure to discuss with your doctor which type of ablation technique they prefer and what might work best for you.

A radio frequency ablation (RFA) is one of the most common forms of endometrial ablation. It is a minimally invasive procedure that is a hybrid between hysteroscopy and the ultrasound-based energy procedures HIFU and MRgFUS.

- *How it works:* Here is what to expect from an RFA. First, your doctor will take a peek inside the uterus with a hysteroscopy. They are checking to confirm that you have FIGO class 0, 1, or 2 fibroids in this compartment of the uterus. If these are present, we are going to remove them first so that the lining of your uterus is returned to its proper state—without fibroids—which will offer a better ablation process. After confirming that the inside of the uterus is normal, your doctor will then insert the ablation special handpiece through the cervix and into the uterus. This handpiece is connected to a machine that sends a radio frequency current to the lining of the endometrium that will heat up and destroy both the superficial and deep layers of the endometrial lining.

Outside of radio frequency, other ablation treatment methods include circulating heated or cooled fluid, water vapor, or a combination of techniques to damage the endometrial lining. Devices and techniques can go in and out of fashion and are dependent on what your doctor is familiar with so you should discuss the method your doctor prefers and uses. The goal across all these technologies is the same: to penetrate both layers of the endometrium with the intention of disabling their ability to regenerate. These techniques have become popular because they are easy to use, relatively safe, require minimal downtime and offer good early results for patients—even if in the future it means you may need or choose additional treatment.

Who's a Good Candidate?

The success (or failure) of an ablation really relies on choosing the right person for the procedure. It's like picking the right tool for the project—for example, you would not use a hammer to screw in a bolt.

So, what makes you a good fit?

- **You're done with childbearing:** Pregnancy is a big no-no after an ablation as we have purposely damaged important layers of the endometrium that can impact a pregnancy. So, if you plan to have kids this is not the procedure for you.
- **You have a normal-size uterus (i.e., pear-shaped, less than 10 to 11 centimeters):** Depending on the type of ablation, the handheld device will only function if the device can fit securely inside the uterus. On the contrary, fluid-based ablations will not work if the size of the uterus is too large to maintain the temperature and pressure inside the uterus required for the ablation to occur.
- **You have tried other treatments:** If you have declined, tried and failed, or do not want major surgical management like a hysterectomy, this may be a good middle ground.

Pros and Cons

Overall, an endometrial ablation is a quick and relatively safe procedure. While bleeding after an ablation is possible, it is rare and occurs only about 2.4 percent of the time. Even less likely is the risk of infection which occurs in less than 2 percent of patients. Your doctor will also discuss something called uterine perforation—when a small hole is made in the uterus—as a potential complication during this procedure. While this understandably sounds scary, it is very rare at around 1.5 percent.

You will be repeatedly counseled that an ablation is not contraception. Even though the goal is to damage the layers that support pregnancy, pregnancy can still occur after an ablation. If you do become pregnant, you're at risk for serious pregnancy complications such as ectopic pregnancy, preterm birth, growth restriction, and postpartum hemorrhage. These types of pregnancies can be complicated so please use contraception after this procedure. Make sure you and your doctor have discussed a backup plan to prevent pregnancy if you are still of reproductive age.

The good news is that according to the data, most people report being really satisfied with their ablation. Satisfaction rates range from 77 to 96 percent and if you are hoping to stop your period entirely, also known as amenorrhea, your chances are around 14 to 70 percent. By twelve months many patients report a significant improvement in their quality of life. That said, there are always outliers and about 5 to 17 percent of women may need a repeat ablation or a hysterectomy later on.

Recovery

The recovery from an ablation is similar to the recovery from a dilation and curettage. You will be released from the ambulatory surgical center on the same day to recover in the comfort of your home. It is common to feel a little crampy or sore in your lower abdominal area, almost as if you did a million crunches. This is nothing that a heating pad, over-the-counter medication, and your most comfortable sweatpants can't handle. You may also have some watery, light pink discharge for the next few days to weeks which is also very common. Make sure you have light pads (not tampons) available until the discharge has resolved. If your discharge has a foul-smelling odor, you should notify your doctor.

If you're experiencing heavy bleeding not caused by structural issues like fibroids, have tried and failed medication options, and are looking for an alternative to hysterectomy, endometrial ablation could be a great option to explore.

Endometrial Ablation vs. Hormonal IUD: Two Paths to Lighter Bleeding

Endometrial ablation techniques are often compared to hormonal IUDs because both options significantly reduce abnormal bleeding. While some studies suggest more IUD users go on to have an ablation or eventually even a hysterectomy as the next step in managing bleeding, there are still key reasons to consider a hormonal IUD before pursuing an ablation or hysterectomy.

The first is that the hormonal IUD will not compromise fertility and also doubles as contraception—a two-for-one benefit. It can also be easily inserted while you are in the office, eliminating the need for anesthesia. However, a potential downside (although not a deal-breaker in my opinion) is the need to replace the IUD if bleeding returns, which may happen around the five-year mark of use.

In contrast the ablation does not provide contraception, requires anesthesia, and the effects on the uterus are irreversible if you desire to become pregnant. For these reasons, it is important to weigh the pros and cons of each option to make the best decision for your lifestyle, health, and reproduction.

Abdominal Myomectomy

Unlike a hysteroscopy where we access the fibroids through your cervix, this is the first method we'll discuss that approaches fibroids from your abdomen. Let's break it down.

- *The setup:* In an open or abdominal myomectomy, a single incision on the abdomen is used to meet, greet, and remove your fibroids. Your doctor might suggest an abdominal myomectomy instead of a less invasive option if your fibroids are large, hard to reach, or in a tricky location in your abdomen. This approach typically means your fibroids are in the muscle (FIGO 2 to 5) or on the surface of your uterus (FIGO 5, 6, 7) and an abdominal incision is the best way to access and remove them. Ultimately, the decision to proceed with this more invasive surgery depends on your comfort and treatment goals.

- *How it works:* An abdominal myomectomy can be performed in a few ways. The most common incision for an abdominal myomectomy is called a "bikini cut" or Pfannenstiel incision—think of an incision made for a cesarean section—low and hidden beneath your underwear. Another option, a midline incision, runs up and down the middle of your abdomen giving your surgeon the best view of your uterus and access to the rest of your abdomen. This isn't very common these days, and is usually reserved for bigger, more complicated cancer cases or a very large uterus.

An open myomectomy may be a little "old school," but it is still the most common abdominal approach for removing fibroids from the uterus. You should be aware, however, that there are less invasive methods available, namely, laparoscopic or robotic-assisted abdominal myomectomy. Both involve smaller incisions distributed in different locations on your abdomen like your belly button. Surgical instruments are inserted through ports in your navel, including a camera that projects a high-definition view of your internal organs on a television screen. Other long surgical instruments are directed into your abdomen to access the uterus. During laparoscopic surgery, your surgeon stands next to your body with these instruments in their hands to remove the fibroids. In a robotic-assisted abdominal myomectomy, the surgeon sits at a console station in the operating room and directs the instruments, which are attached to a robotic operative system positioned near your body.

What Happens Next: Myomectomy Step-by-Step

Once your surgeon is inside your abdomen, open myomectomies and laparoscopic myomectomies are not very different. Let's walk through the steps together. For an abdominal myomectomy, the uterus is lifted out of your abdomen and brought through your skin incision. It is never detached from your body. In laparoscopic procedures the uterus remains entirely in the abdomen. The tools work through small incisions.

First, it's picture time. I always take a few snapshots of a patient's pelvis, including the fallopian tubes and ovaries, so they can see what is going on in their body. You can ask your surgeon to do the same if you're not squeamish. Doing so will give you a full visual of what is going on inside your belly and reinforce the decision you made was the best for your body. Next, it's time to mentally map out the safest way to remove fibroids in a way that minimizes incisions on your uterus, avoids the organs around your uterus—including your bladder, intestines, and major blood vessels—and minimizes blood loss.

Before starting, your surgeon will use a few tricks to help minimize blood loss. This can range all the way from injecting a medication directly into the fibroids to constrict blood vessels, to wrapping a tourniquet around major blood vessels to the uterus. From here, your surgeon will determine where to make incisions on the uterus that maximize removing fibroids while minimizing blood loss. Each incision will reveal a fibroid that can then be plucked out of the uterus, leaving a hollow space behind. When the fibroid is removed, we close the remaining, hollow space with suture—a surgical thread—layer by layer, until the space is tightly sealed. This not only will minimize bleeding, it will promote healing of the uterine muscle. We repeat this until all the fibroids are removed and the uterus is sutured back together. In an abdominal myomectomy the uterus is guided back through the skin and into the abdomen. From here, all the layers of the body we open to make our way to the uterus are again closed with suture. During laparoscopy we remove all of the instruments from inside the body, slowly deflate the abdomen that was filled with carbon dioxide gas, and only select layers are closed. Finally, we close your skin incision(s) with sutures—rarely with staples. Voilà, your surgery is done! From here your anesthesiologist will slowly and gently remove the anesthesia and wake you up from surgery.

Pros and Cons of Abdominal Myomectomy: Open vs. Laparoscopic

Making the decision to undergo a major surgery is not something you or I should take lightly. As someone who performs large myomectomies and guides people through this experience, I know it can be challenging. What I can tell you from years of experience is that while recovery can be difficult, the result can be life changing.

Choosing between open and laparoscopic myomectomy is a hot topic in gynecology as there are key benefits to both. Let's discuss both options so you can make the best decision for yourself.

An open myomectomy is potentially beneficial for fibroids that are deeply embedded in the uterus that laparoscopic procedures may miss or not be able to access. The goal of abdominal myomectomy is to remove all visible and palpable fibroids, even those as small as a grain of rice, to ensure thorough treatment. For a complex, multi-fibroid uterus, an open approach provides your surgeon the clearest view of the uterus and nearby organs. And although it may be a more invasive procedure, the blood loss is typically not significantly more than with a laparoscopic procedure.

The recovery is longer than less invasive options, but sometimes when it comes to fibroids and heavy menstrual bleeding it takes a "go big or go home" approach to evict fibroids out of your uterus and hit the reset button on your health. If you've been living with severe bleeding, pain, and pelvic pressure symptoms, the long-term relief the procedure brings can make every bit of your recovery worth it.

A main goal of any myomectomy is to preserve and maintain the integrity of the uterus. Whether you are hoping to maintain your fertility or simply want to keep your uterus, it is our job to help support your decision. It is not often that we enter the operating room with the plan of performing a myomectomy (either open or laparoscopic) and end up with an unplanned hysterectomy. When I explain this to patients, I ask them to think of their uterus as a puzzle. During a myomectomy we are taking twenty pieces out of a hundred-piece puzzle. A majority of the time, after we have completed removing those pieces, we are able to recreate a puzzle that looks and will function like a uterus. In very rare instances, however, if too many pieces are removed or if large pieces are removed, the uterus may become impossible to salvage.

When Bleeding Happens

During your informed consent process, we should always review the risk of bleeding during surgery. With any myomectomy, bleeding can be significant hence the many safeguards we put in place to anticipate and reduce bleeding. Unfortunately, another reason for an unplanned hysterectomy is if bleeding cannot be controlled despite medication and other surgical efforts. Your uterus is supplied by a superhighway of blood vessels that start at the top and run down to the bottom of the uterus. Surgery on the uterus is knowingly a bloody business. If bleeding becomes quick and severe, it can be challenging to control and may pose a life-threatening risk to your health. Your doctor may have to make the tough call to remove your uterus to stop the bleeding and save your life. Remember and be reassured, this scenario is very rare. We respect your decision to keep your uterus and will do everything possible to honor that desire.

Nobody Wants a Scar: The Small Price for Big Relief

Many of my patients are concerned about scarring and rightfully so— our skin is often the first reflection of health and it is appropriate to be concerned about aesthetics. With an open myomectomy, your incision will sit low on your abdomen, just below your underwear in a discreet location, and is generally just slightly larger than your uterus. Often your surgeon can estimate the anticipated size of the incision for you so there will not be any surprises. Robotic surgery involves at least three to four incisions across the middle part of the abdomen, while laparoscopy usually uses three to four incisions below the belly button. In both laparoscopy and robotics, one of the smaller incisions is usually extended in size (either at the belly button or just above the pubic line) to facilitate taking the fibroids out of the abdomen.

Depending on how your skin heals, and how you dress, scars can be visible for years. It is also worth considering how these visible scars and incisions may impact your self-esteem. These concerns and the location of the incisions should definitely be discussed with your surgeon. If you have richly melanated skin (e.g., of African, Hispanic, or Asian descent) you should also discuss the possibility of developing keloid scars. Keloids are thick, raised scars that extend beyond the original incision site and can occur after skin injury like surgery. Your tendency to form scars or keloids may influence your decision about the distribution of incisions. We will discuss how to optimize your healing more in Chapter 12.

Naturally, small incisions mean a shorter or no hospital stay at all. With laparoscopic procedures patients are typically sent home the same day, as recovery from smaller incisions is quicker and the procedure is less invasive. In contrast, patients having abdominal myomectomies are typically admitted to the hospital for typically two and no more than three days. The primary reason for this is due to the larger incisions, and the resulting need for IV and oral pain relief after a more invasive procedure. So, while laparoscopic procedures will get you home and back on your feet much sooner, discuss with your surgeon if the abdominal approach for a more complex case including the extra time spent in the hospital and for recovery is worth it.

Laparoscopic Radio Frequency Ablation (RFA): A Minimally Invasive Option for Fibroid Treatment

For those looking to address fibroids while avoiding a hysterectomy, laparoscopic radio frequency ablation (RFA) offers an innovative marriage between RFA technology and minimally invasive laparoscopy.

In this procedure, a small incision is made on the abdomen, much like in traditional laparoscopy. A specialized RFA device is used to deliver controlled radio frequency energy directly to FIGO class 2 to 7 fibroids, effectively destroying the fibroid tissue while sparing healthy uterine tissue.

This targeted approach provides several advantages:

- *Precision: Direct treatment of fibroids with minimal impact on surrounding tissue.*
- *Minimally invasive: Smaller incisions lead to reduced pain and quicker recovery.*
- *Rapid return to daily life: Most patients experience shorter downtime and faster healing.*

Laparoscopic RFA is an excellent alternative for people who are done with childbearing but seek alternative fibroid treatment without undergoing more invasive surgical procedures.

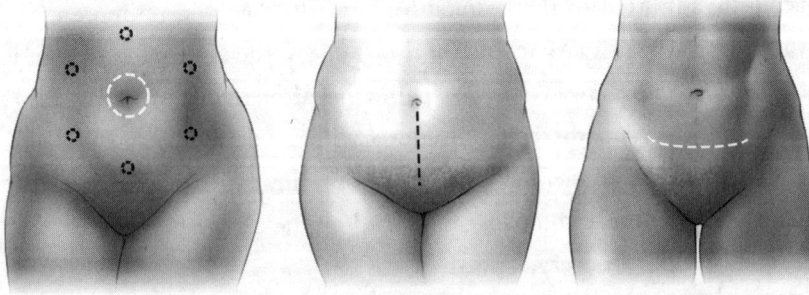

Laparoscopic   **Vertical line**   **Transverse line**

From Surgery to Stork: Fertility and Pregnancy After Myomectomy

Several studies show that for most patients, infertility improves after myomectomy, especially if fibroids are thought to be the primary reason for infertility. Submucosal fibroids and multiple large fibroids indeed have a negative impact on fertility rates, but many studies note that after a myomectomy fertility rates can increase by 50 to 70 percent. Even if you are unsure of your fertility goals, it is crucial to discuss with your doctor how surgery on your uterus can impact your ability to conceive and how extensive uterine surgery could influence how you deliver your future children.

While a myomectomy—either open or laparoscopic—can positively influence your fertility, the bigger reason for this conversation is because opinions regarding the safest delivery route (vaginal versus planned C-section) after a myomectomy can be controversial for obstetricians and gynecologists. Normally, if you've had a myomectomy, we recommend a planned cesarean delivery as early as thirty-seven weeks. You may ask, "Well, what is the big deal?" I have an answer for that. Your obstetrician is concerned about the risk of uterine rupture, which is an unexpected and potentially devastating opening of the uterus muscle during pregnancy or labor. A uterine rupture can be detrimental for a pregnancy—in many cases it is life-threatening for the mother—often leading to heavy bleeding or even hysterectomy.

Although backed by limited data, the risk of uterine rupture varies from .4 to 1.7 percent after an abdominal myomectomy and .49 to 1.2 percent after a laparoscopic myomectomy. Admittedly this risk seems statistically low but when considering the grave consequences of a uterine rupture, many obstetricians—especially those who have seen and managed a uterine rupture—are not willing to take this risk for you or your pregnancy. On average your obstetrician will quote a risk of 1 percent but this is likely not an accurate estimate for a few reasons. One, because most patients do elect for a scheduled C-section given our current guidelines and two, uterine ruptures following a myomectomy are not centrally reported. This prevents tracking to analyze and gather data on the true risk of uterine rupture in pregnancy or during labor on someone with a prior myomectomy.

The root of this concern stems from older, limited data suggesting that if the endometrial cavity (the space where the pregnancy grows) is opened during surgery the risk of uterine rupture was as high as 2.5 percent. Over time obstetricians have extended this recommendation to what is our true concern, which is the impact of removing large fibroids or fibroids at the top of the uterus. This core concern is based on the concept that the muscle-scar combination that fills the repaired defect does not heal to its presurgery strength and the intense force of labor could disrupt these areas causing a catastrophic uterine rupture.

To date, we don't have any solid studies to guide recommendations regarding vaginal delivery versus elective scheduled C-sections. Why? Because there are so many factors that influence decision-making including:

- Number, size, and location of fibroids removed
- Number of incisions made in the uterus
- Type of suture used and number of layers used to close the space left behind

And this is just the tip of the iceberg of considerations that come to mind when making these important recommendations.

Unfortunately, the real risk of uterine rupture after a myomectomy remains unknown, so you should be prepared to be counseled that after a laparoscopic or open myomectomy you may be advised to have a cesarean section for the delivery of your future children. Your doctor will typically note this recommendation in your operative report—the official play-by-play of your surgery—and you should plan to have a verbal conversation about this issue before and after your surgery.

Like any recommendation, your plan for delivery has to be personalized to your specific needs and the experience of your surgeon, and the comfort of your obstetrician—if they are not the same person. For instance, there have been cases where I have removed very superficial pedunculated (FIGO 0, 1, 6, 7) fibroids and felt completely comfortable moving forward with a vaginal delivery in these same patients. But remember, this conversation and recommendation will happen on a case-by-case basis based on your unique circumstance.

If you are not open to the idea of two major surgeries—one surgery now and another later—then perhaps a myomectomy is not for you. Don't worry, you have options, and your surgeon can continue to guide you toward a decision that aligns with your desire to have children, health goals, and lifestyle.

If you are amenable to the role of myomectomy as a part of your fertility plan and understand the potential for future surgery, there is one more ask and that is to wait a minimum of six months after surgery before trying to conceive. This allows the uterus to optimize healing and reduce the risk of complications such as uterine rupture or an abnormal attachment of the placenta to the uterus. A little patience is all we ask and goes a long way to ensure a smoother journey ahead.

Recovery

If you are bouncing between the pros and cons of an open myomectomy versus a laparoscopic (or robotic) procedure, a major factor to consider is the recovery period. Recovery from an open myomectomy versus laparoscopic/robotic myomectomy will not be the same. In general, the recovery from an open myomectomy is often a bit longer at around 4 to 6 weeks. You'll have to take more time off work compared to laparoscopic or robotic procedures. The larger incision concentrated on your lower abdomen may almost certainly come with a little more discomfort as you start to get back into the groove of life. If your tolerance for pain or discomfort isn't on the high end, you may need to take medication for longer than what is typical with a laparoscopic procedure. Think of this recovery as a marathon and definitely not a sprint. You need to pace yourself during your four-to-six-week recovery and let your body heal one day at a time. There should be no heavy lifting or strenuous exercise—including sex or driving—until you are off any strong medications and feel well enough to react quickly. Most patients, however, do feel significantly better at their two-week postoperative visit. The key is to listen to your body and allow yourself to rest and heal.

Now, on the other hand, if your lifestyle or even personal preference is for a quick snap back, then perhaps you should focus on a laparoscopic or robotic procedure. Smaller incisions spread across your abdomen tend to lead to a quicker recovery, and you can often return to work, exercise, and everything else you love sooner. Even with the potential for a faster recovery—most people feel well enough to return to work in 2 to 3 weeks—your minimally invasive recovery is still not a sprint, but perhaps a brisk walk. You will need to slow down and listen to your body.

Charting Your Own Path

I hope you now have a clearer road map of both the minimally and moderately invasive treatment options that may be available to you before you consider a hysterectomy, including a general understanding of how each treatment varies in invasiveness, recovery, and effectiveness in treating bleeding, pain, or pelvic pressure. Surgery—even single day ambulatory options—can feel intimidating and overwhelming, but if the medical treatments you have tried have not worked to sufficiently manage your symptoms, it may be time to move on to the next step of care. We have covered a lot here from more simple procedures like a dilation and curettage and uterine artery embolization, to more invasive procedures like open and laparoscopic myomectomy.

The goal of all this is to demystify your options and help you make informed and empowered decisions without the fear of procedures, surgery and recovery holding you back. This is how you regain control of your health. Understanding the differences in recovery time, risks, benefits, alternatives, and potential complications will help you make a decision that aligns with your immediate and long-term health goals, fertility, and comfort level.

8

Gender-Affirming Hysterectomy

I spend a good portion of my time with patients focused on the physical problems the uterus and ovaries can contribute to like fibroids, pelvic pain, and endometriosis. As a result, I often consider hysterectomies when something is physically wrong with your uterus and removing it is one way to fix it. Yet your decision to proceed with a hysterectomy may be more nuanced than that. Your goal may be greater peace and comfort with yourself and your body. While this can be incredibly liberating, it also raises its own set of questions and concerns.

For too long now the medical community has not been a good advocate for gender-affirming medical care—and it has caused countless people to suffer. As the medical field moves toward greater advocacy for the transgender and nonbinary communities, increased effort has been made to correct the injustice suffered by these communities in their medical experience. We have started to listen, and a collaborative community of doctors and others in the medical field have begun to rally around the medical, surgical, psychological, financial, and sociocultural needs of those seeking gender-affirming care. What has come out of this are still-evolving but clearer steps to help those seeking gender-affirming hysterectomies manage the stress, depression, and anxiety that may come with living with gender dysphoria, including clear treatment and surgical options that align your mental and physical needs. This chapter will help you navigate those steps from the perspective of both gynecological care more broadly, and hysterectomy specifically.

There is not a clear number of how many transgender men or nonbinary people undergo hysterectomy surgery each year. At this time of this writing, it is believed to be less than 1 percent of all hysterectomies. This number is rapidly growing as access to surgery is improving and the stress caused by gender dysphoria is becoming more understood. Of the transgender and nonbinary patients who have had a hysterectomy, well over a half cite their gender identity concerns as the main reason for the decision to proceed with a hysterectomy. They also report a high level of satisfaction with their surgery and rarely regret it. In another study, 37 percent of respondents have a hysterectomy to avoid future gynecological appointments. This is an indication that for a significant number of people, gynecological care has the potential to be very traumatic. This is a signal to physicians and the larger medical community that we have to listen, be present, and do better for our transgender and gender-fluid patients.

Gender-affirming medical care usually centers around two things: gender-affirming hormonal therapy (GAHT), commonly called hormone replacement therapy (HRT), and gender-affirming surgery (GAS). GAHT uses hormones like testosterone and estrogen blockers to help you develop more masculine physical characteristics in line with your gender identity. Several guidelines are available to help manage the facial, vocal, and physical transition from a female to male. GAS is any surgery, including removal of the breast tissue, uterus, fallopian tubes, and ovaries, that aims to align your physical appearance with your identity. However, while GAHT and GAS are now the standard of care for patients undergoing their transition and thought to be medically necessary for patients undergoing transition, transgender and nonbinary patients are not a monolith. You may or may not opt for hormonal treatment or surgery—you may opt for one and not the other. You get to decide, and you deserve to have a trusted partner in your doctor when making these decisions. The decisions that you make are important and life changing. You don't have to make all the decisions at once and you don't have to do everything all at once. You are unique, and you have options with how you go through this process. You get to align every part of your transition with your sense of self.

The process of a hysterectomy is the same for trans men and nonbinary people as it is for cisgender women. A hysterectomy remains the removal of the uterus, with or without the removal of the cervix. Similar to cisgender women, the route of hysterectomy can take place by a few approaches—open, laparoscopic, robotic, and perhaps even vaginal—based on the size of your uterus, features of your body, and other planned surgeries. When hysterectomy alone is performed, the complication rates are no different from the experiences of cisgender women. Complication rates can increase when other genital surgeries are combined, but generally these are safe surgeries. However, there is a lot that we know and do not know about the unique situation of surgery in the context of hormonal therapy, and there are special questions you may want to ask. It is important that you know and understand the full landscape of questions, concerns, and limitations on medical knowledge so that you can make empowered decisions with your body and your life.

First Priority: Finding Your Care Team

If you're in the transgender and nonbinary communities, it's probably not news to you that engaging with the medical profession is often fraught with challenges, judgment, and stigma. For far too long, the gender-affirming journey for transgender and nonbinary people has been marked by significant mental health stigma. Mental health providers and physicians have pathologized your experience—for years, people in transition were subjected to years of forced psychiatric evaluations to determine whether their gender dysphoria was real and if their experience was sufficient enough to warrant gender-affirming treatment. These medical loopholes discouraged engagement with the medical community. We used these tactics to delay or restrict necessary treatment to these patients. While the medical profession is changing and improving a lot, it can still be hard to find affirming care providers. It may take some time and effort on your part, but it's important to assemble a good team. A medical team that is knowledgeable and supportive of your decision is key as you navigate this process.

To help support your decision-making process, look for physicians who are comfortable with informed consent. The informed consent model supports your autonomy in making decisions that are in the best interest of your body. Sounds basic, right? Well, things were not always this way. It is a far departure from the assumption that gender dysphoria is a mental health illness and that we—the doctors—know what is best for you. But a provider who practices informed consent will firmly position you as the expert of your physical, social, and emotional needs. It rejects the separate standards and unnecessary hurdles that transgender and nonbinary people have and continue to face. The informed consent model allows you and your healthcare team to individualize your care based on the standard guidelines used for all patients regardless of their gender. This means that your care team will provide unbiased, medically accurate information to help you make a decision about every step of your transition. From hormone use to the decision to have a hysterectomy, you will be given the tools and understanding of the short- and long-term risks of the decisions you make that may impact your medical or mental healthcare over your lifespan. At the core, you get to be you. There is not one way to do a gender transition, this process is about you. You can simply ask any providers you meet with if they practice informed consent.

I confess that I often cringe when patients say, "I googled [insert issue]" because you never know what you are going to dredge up from the depths of the internet. But this is a unique situation so I'm going to suggest that a Google search can be a great place to start to help you find a gender-affirming care team. First you can search the provider directory of organizations that are committed to access and providing gender-affirming care to patients. Current and leading organizations that you may consider include WPATH (World Professional Association for Transgender Health); GLMA (Health Professionals Advancing LGBTQ Equality); and OutCare Health (a nationwide health resource for LGBTQ+ healthcare). You can also use keywords to help narrow your search to find a healthcare team, such as:

- trans-friendly doctor near me
- LGBTQ medical care
- gender-affirming care near me
- WPATH provider near me
- LGBTQ+ community center (often great resources for everything from surgeons to gynecologists to therapists and much more)

You should simultaneously be gathering information from your insurance provider. Insurance can be a huge hurdle in the process, though slowly things are getting better. In any case, your provider's website and customer service representatives can be a resource for information about everything from providers to what, if anything, is covered. You can search the provider directory on the insurance website. Many medical providers can choose to promote their comfort with gender-affirming care by using phrases such as *LGBTQ+* or *trans-affirming care* in their byline. Care providers can also detail any additional or special training in gender-affirming care they have, the types of gender-confirming treatments they offer, and how long they have been caring for trans people.

You are also going to want to better understand your benefit coverage for your transition. Historically, most current transition surgeries are paid for out of pocket; any insurance coverage will be minimal. This is finally changing thanks to the amazing advocacy of transgender and nonbinary health advocates, but it is unfortunately not for all insurances or for all surgeries. So, you'll want to know what's covered and what's not. You'll also want to know if there are any prior authorizations, committees, selection criteria, physicians' notes, or other hurdles you'll have to manage in order to receive the surgery (or surgeries) you require covered. It is best to explore this ahead of time so that you and your healthcare team can tackle these hurdles head-on together and not have any surprises that can derail your journey.

As you navigate the web of insurance it is important to keep a track of your conversations and interactions with your insurance company. Like the kids say, you need to keep receipts. Every conversation with them should be documented so that from one agent to the next the criteria that is required does not get changed. After each phone call you can ask for the call number and the first name and last initial of the representative you spoke with. This will be especially important if they try to deny the insurance claims that you make in the future.

It will involve some work on your part, but after you find your care team and know where things stand with your coverage, the heavy lifting is really going to be on us. This means you will find a team well versed in hormone therapy and be better able to weigh the pros and cons of decisions like keeping your uterus, ovaries, or cervix, experts to help explore your fertility, psychologists to help manage your mental health, and more! Finding a good team is important; it's our job to make sure you understand the definitive nature of your decisions and then respect whatever decision you make. We provide you context and options while you make decisions that align with your values and spirit.

Important Questions to Consider

The decisions you make along your gender-affirming journey are not the same for everyone. The intersection of gender identity and human biology is undoubtedly complex, and it may take several discussions with a multidisciplinary team to work through all the different aspects that come up. There are some fundamental questions you may want to consider, however, before you start or continue your journey. Things like:

- Do I need to remove my uterus if I want to avoid surgery altogether?
- What is the current data to support my decision?
- How do I navigate my transition if I still have or want to keep my biologically female reproductive organs?
- Do I need to perform all gender-affirming surgery as a part of my transition, or do I have the freedom to choose which procedures are right for me?
- What should I consider if I think I may want to keep my ovaries?
- What are my options if I may want to consider pregnancy one day?

This is only the tip of the iceberg, but no worries. Your trained, multidisciplinary team will walk you through this and concerns you may have not even considered well before any surgical decisions are made.

Removing the Uterus and Ovaries: Pros and Cons

Let's start with what we know about the pros of removing the uterus and ovaries. Removal of the uterus is associated with a significant improvement of gender dysphoria. It's the standard of care and considered deemed medically necessary for patients undergoing transition because the data and lived experience on this is so strong. As a result, there are more centers of excellence available to guide you. There is also growing insurance coverage and legal protection to support your transition.

We also know that without these structures there is a significant decrease in ovarian, fallopian tubes, uterine, and cervical cancers. Removing them also eliminates the stress of menstruation and the need for regular gynecological visits for Pap smears.

Your risk-benefit analysis should also consider reasons to keep your uterus. For starters, keeping the uterus and ovaries avoids a surgical procedure and an abdominal scar. A scar might not seem like a big deal, but it can remind you of your transition on a daily basis. It can provoke unsolicited questions regarding the scar(s) that you may or may not be ready to address. Thankfully, new minimally invasive surgery options can keep scarring to a minimum.

We don't know all the long-term effects of testosterone on the uterus and ovaries but if you choose to keep your uterus, you will likely stop menstruating. If you do still have an occasional period, there are options to stop bleeding, including long-term contraception, hormonal IUDs, or an endometrial ablation. Revisit Chapters 3 and 4 if you need a refresher on these. It may seem obvious, but keeping your uterus and ovaries preserves your fertility and you should also take a moment to consider that. In practice, the data suggests that very few transgender men carry a pregnancy and/or use their preserved eggs after gender-affirming treatment but you should know this is an option. Have you considered the potential for having children in the future? Have you ever had the thought of carrying a pregnancy? Do you have any interest in preserving your eggs even if you do not want to carry a pregnancy yourself? Consider both your short- or long-term goals—is it worth keeping your uterus and ovaries in order to have biological children and then explore surgery after you are done having children? Or is it more important to you to have surgery now?

Some trans men and nonbinary patients have their uteruses removed but keep their ovaries. One of the main reasons they do so is their potential desire to have children, but it's important to know that taking testosterone as part of your GAHT will also impact your fertility. There is no clear protocol for fertility treatments after you have started GAHT except that most times it does require you to stop your testosterone treatment. The upside is that the fertility options available to you do not differ from cisgender people. Depending on your desires, the options for egg freezing, embryo preservation, sperm donation, a gestational carrier, and even adoption should be discussed as a way to help you build your family if you decide. The option to remove the ovaries and store them for future use, also called ovarian preservation, is experimental but will hopefully be the standard of care and widely available over time. Hormonal management, fertility, and childbearing have numerous psychological, legal, and medical moving parts. I recommend patients discuss their concerns with a reproductive endocrinologist and infertility specialist, also known as an REI doctor. They can help you understand the nuances of your fertility options as they can vary by age, state, and insurance.

Risks Associated with Removing Your Ovaries

If you are taking testosterone as part of your transition, and you decide to keep your ovaries, you should know that researchers are still working to understand the impact of long-term testosterone therapy on the uterus and the ovaries. Under a microscope, testosterone changes what the ovaries look like. We see an increase in testosterone receptors that make the ovaries look similar to a condition known as polycystic ovarian syndrome (PCOS). Cisgender women with PCOS have an increased risk of ovarian and uterine cancer. While this is all theoretical, there is a concern that this could lead to an increased risk of ovarian and possibly uterine cancer in trans men and nonbinary people who choose to keep their ovaries. Right now, we simply do not have an answer to assess this risk. What we do know is that for cisgender women the ovaries are very important. The estrogens and other hormones the ovaries make are not only key to a healthy heart, bones, and brain, but also to your overall quality of life. When a cisgender woman removes her ovaries before the age of forty-five to fifty we know that her risk of death increases, especially from cardiovascular disease and dementia. We would expect that most trans men would have their ovaries removed around this time or earlier. While we cannot extrapolate what happens to cisgender women without ovaries to transgender men with or without ovaries on testosterone therapy, this is a serious consideration you should discuss with your healthcare team.

A Gender-Affirming Hysterectomy: Your Path, Your Choice

As you consider a gender-affirming hysterectomy, it's important to acknowledge that this decision is deeply personal and, at times, complex. The surgery can bring immense relief by aligning your body more closely with your gender identity, reducing gender dysphoria, and eliminating the need for menstruation-related care. For many, this step offers a sense of peace and empowerment. However, it's equally important to weigh the potential challenges—surgical risks, changes in hormone balance, and the emotional impact of this transition.

Testosterone therapy can continue to play a vital role in your journey, enhancing your comfort in your body and supporting your well-being post-hysterectomy. But, keeping your ovaries or removing them entirely is a decision worth careful thought. Retaining your ovaries can help maintain hormone production and reduce long-term health risks associated with bone density and cardiovascular health, especially if you prefer a more gradual hormonal shift. However, removing them may provide relief from hormonal cycles that could still be trigger menstruation or other menstrual-related symptoms.

Most importantly, finding a medical team that respects and understands your goals is essential. Take your time to surround yourself with professionals who listen, respect your identity, and guide you through this process with care and empathy. You deserve to feel seen and supported every step of the way, making decisions that are not only right for your body but for your sense of self.

9

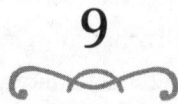

Hysterectomy 101

The Ultimate Guide to Choosing Your
Uterus's Exit Strategy

Wen patients come to my office and say, "I had a hysterectomy" I often have to probe a little bit to understand what they mean. Often, I hear things like, "They took everything out," or, "I had a partial hysterectomy," and sometimes even "I don't know, I just know I don't bleed anymore." These conversations have taught me that the word *hysterectomy* means different things to different people regardless if you are the patient or the doctor. This chapter is all about getting us on the same page about what a hysterectomy is and is not. A hysterectomy is not a one-size-fits-all procedure and can vary from person to person based on two points:

1. What exactly are we removing? Is it only the uterus, or are you also have the cervix removed? Also, are you removing the ovaries and/or fallopian tubes?
2. How is the uterus being removed? What method or approach is going to be used to remove the uterus? Will it be from the vagina,

a single, long incision, or several small incisions on the abdomen as with laparoscopy?

Once you understand these basics you and your doctor will have a reference point from which all other conversations can flow.

Patients are often appropriately concerned about safety, how long the recovery will be, and how we can minimize scarring. As a surgeon, I also share your concerns about safety, but also consider operating time as a means to reduce complications based on your surgical and medical conditions. We need to consider past medical history like C-sections, other abdominal surgeries, endometriosis which might influence scar tissue, the size of your uterus, the location of fibroids, your ability to tolerate anesthesia and your overall health. All of this shapes how we approach decisions about your surgery.

By having these conversations and basic understanding, we are making sure that your needs and my medical expertise are aligned. This way we can approach your surgery in a way that feels right for you—with safety and outcome in mind.

I Am Having a Hysterectomy: Coming to Terms with What Is Being Removed

There are several terms you will hear to describe a hysterectomy; they refer to what exactly is being removed. If you are not familiar with these terms, it can be a little overwhelming. When you discuss your surgery with your healthcare team it is important that you and your surgeon speak the same language. These are the terms you need to understand when considering a hysterectomy:

- **Subtotal (or supracervical) hysterectomy:** A subtotal, supracervical, or what some doctors and patients call a partial hysterectomy, involves the removal of the top part of the uterus, also known as the body, and leaves behind the cervix, ovaries, or fallopian

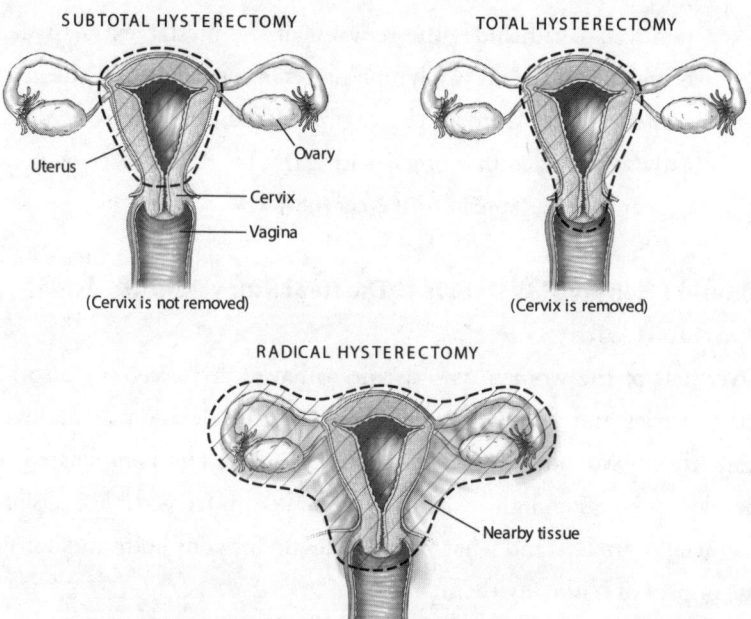

SUBTOTAL HYSTERECTOMY

Uterus
Ovary
Cervix
Vagina

(Cervix is not removed)

TOTAL HYSTERECTOMY

(Cervix is removed)

RADICAL HYSTERECTOMY

Nearby tissue

tubes. This surgery will address where most fibroids, adenomyosis, and heavy bleeding originates. After this procedure you will not be able to get pregnant because the main part of your uterus is removed. Occasionally a small amount of bleeding or spotting is possible if some endometrial tissue is in or near the cervix.

- **Total hysterectomy:** A total hysterectomy is when we remove the entire uterus along with the cervix, the lower portion of the uterus. Like a subtotal hysterectomy, this term only addresses the uterus and has nothing to do with the management of the ovaries or fallopian tubes.

- **Simple hysterectomy:** This refers to the extent of your surgery, or how much tissue is being removed. The term "simple" implies only the uterus is removed and no extra tissue on either side of the uterus is removed. This is the most common type of hysterectomy performed worldwide.

- **Radical hysterectomy:** A radical hysterectomy is a more extensive procedure. Radical refers to the need to have additional tissue removed—it includes the removal of the uterus, extra tissue on both sides of the uterus, lymph nodes in the pelvis near the uterus, and the upper third of the vagina. A radical hysterectomy typically takes place in women with early cervical cancer or uterine cancer that has spread to the cervix.

Should I Remove My Ovaries? The Real Story Behind Ovarian Health

Over half of the women who decide to have a hysterectomy also have their ovaries and fallopian tubes removed. The decision to remove or keep these two hormonal powerhouses removed is complicated and should not be taken lightly. Before you make this irreversible decision, it is crucial to understand what your ovaries do for your body and consider the impact of removing them.

Let's start with the basics: If you recall our earlier anatomy lesson, your ovaries are a pair of small, almond-shaped organs on either side of the uterus. Together they are the foundation of your hormonal and reproductive health. Beyond being the home for your eggs, the ovaries are also the primary source of the most important female reproductive hormones: estrogen, progesterone, and testosterone. Estrogen, in particular, is critical not only to your reproductive health but also to your heart, brain, and bone health. So, it is easy to understand why removing your ovaries can be such a big decision.

Key reasons you might want to consider keeping your ovaries:

- **Avoiding early menopause:** Menopause starts when you have gone one full year with no period. Leading up to and after menopause, the ovaries significantly decrease their production of estrogen leading to hot flashes, trouble sleeping, mood swings, brain fog, and low libido. In the United States the average age of menopause in the US is fifty to fifty-two for white women, but can range from forty-five to fifty-eight years old—primarily influenced by ethnicity and socioeconomic factors. We do not have a crystal ball to know when you will start menopause, but removing your ovaries will immediately signal a drop in estrogen leading to sudden and intense hot flashes. Other symptoms may follow soon after.

- **Bone health:** Estrogen is critical to maintaining bone health. It prevents the weakening of bones which can lead to osteoporosis, a condition where bones become fragile and are more likely to break. Women with their ovaries or women on HRT are at lower risk for osteoporosis. As you age, maintaining strong bones is important to decrease your risk of back, hip, or wrist fractures.

- **Cardiovascular health:** Estrogen is known to have a protective effect on the heart, helping to reduce your risk of heart disease. This protective effect decreases as women enter menopause, and studies show that women without ovaries have higher rates of heart disease; removing both ovaries before the age of forty-five is associated with an increased risk of death from heart disease. With cardiovascular disease being an overall leading cause of death in women, it is important to assess your risk, and if you are a candidate for hormone replacement therapy to replace the estrogen you lose without ovaries.

- **Mental health:** Research suggests that removing the ovaries before natural menopause can increase the risk of certain neurological diseases like Parkinson's and dementia. A sudden loss of estrogen can contribute to mental health challenges like depression and anxiety. Estrogen plays a protective role in the brain and a sudden decrease can have far reaching effects on your mental health and well-being.

- **Sexual health:** Estrogen is also essential to maintain your sexual health. Over time, the lack of estrogen can decrease your libido and impact vaginal health which can lead to vaginal dryness and discomfort during sex. These changes can cause emotional strain and physical discomfort—both of which can significantly impact your relationship. Maintaining your ovaries or starting hormone replacement therapy may help encourage a healthy sex life and promote healthy vaginal tissue.

- **Overall life expectancy:** Many studies have shown the overall life expectancy of women with their ovaries to be greater than those who have had their ovaries removed. Even if you have an average risk of ovarian cancer, major studies have found that keeping your ovaries until at least age sixty-five can benefit your overall long-term survival.

Estrogen's protective effects on heart, bone, and brain health are key factors in these findings. These risks are compelling enough to convince many women to keep their ovaries. However, there are instances where removing the ovaries should be strongly considered. In fact, for some women, removing their ovaries can provide significant health benefits.

Some key reasons you might want to consider removing your ovaries:

- **High risk for ovarian or breast cancer:** If you have a family history of breast or ovarian cancer or have the BRCA (BReast CAncer) gene mutation, removing your ovaries can significantly decrease your risk of ovarian cancer. The BRCA gene repairs errors in our DNA. If these errors in your DNA are not repaired, cells are able to grow and divide without regulation. When there is no regulation you have an increased risk of developing certain types of cancers—in this case breast, ovarian, and peritoneal (the thin layer of cells that lines the inside of your body). Female members of families with a defective BRCA1/2 gene have a significantly increased risk of breast and ovarian cancer. The current recommendation for BRCA 1 and 2 carriers is that they have a risk-reducing bilateral salpingo-oophorectomy (RRBSO)—removal of the ovaries and fallopian tubes to reduce the risk of developing cancer. A risk-reducing BSO in BRCA 1 carriers is recommended by age thirty to forty years and forty to forty-five years in BRCA2 women who typically have ovarian cancer found later in life. An RR BSO is the only proven intervention to reduce the risk of ovarian cancer upward of 96 percent and breast cancer of up to 50 percent. There are other genetic risks for ovarian cancer. Women who are carriers of BRIP1, RAD51C, RAD51D genes and families with Lynch syndrome (a genetic syndrome with an increased risk of colon, uterine, and ovarian cancer) should also consider an RRBSO at the time of hysterectomy.

- **Severe endometriosis or chronic pelvic pain:** Surgery is not the first line treatment for endometriosis, however if medical management fails, sometimes surgery is necessary to remove endometriotic tissue and restoration of normal anatomy that causes problematic symptoms. Many women with endometriosis undergo multiple surgeries—41 percent of endometriosis patients in fact reported repeat surgeries. In another study, a whooping 93 percent reported three or fewer surgeries. For definitive management, sometimes a hysterectomy along with removal of the ovaries is recommended. Removing the ovaries removes the estrogen that feeds endometriosis implants and therefore improves your pain. Many studies show that removing the ovaries provides greater improvement in pain and quality-of-life scores—this may be something for you to think about.

- **Risk for future ovarian cysts:** Your ovaries will continue to produce hormones such as estrogen, progesterone, and testosterone even after the uterus is removed. The risk of ovarian cancer increases over time, making it the second leading gynecological cancer and the deadliest gynecological cancer. Because the ovaries remain hormonally active there is a possibility of developing an ovarian cyst or mass months to even years after your hysterectomy. In fact, nearly 5 to 8 percent of women will develop ovarian cysts after their hysterectomy with nearly half of these occurring within the first year of surgery. While most of these cysts are non-cancerous, the physical and emotional stress of managing an ovarian cyst should not be underestimated. Additionally, the risk of ovarian cancer can increase with age. If you choose to retain your ovaries you should understand that the potential for ovarian cysts, and cancer masses, remains. If imaging or blood work raises concerns about a cyst or mass, you may need additional testing (blood work and imaging) and in some cases, surgery to rule out cancer. Being aware of this possibility can help you make an informed decision about whether to retain your ovaries.

- **Postmenopausal ovarian masses:** If an ovarian mass is detected after menopause, the risk of it being malignant increases. In these cases, your doctor may recommend removing the ovaries as a precaution to eliminate the risk of ovarian cancer.

A majority of women opt to have their ovaries removed during hysterectomy even if they don't have a family history of cancer. However, it is worth remembering that your ovaries are powerful, not just for your bone, brain, and heart health, but also for your longevity. Make it a point to have an in-depth conversation with your doctor about whether removing your ovaries is in your best interest.

When you talk to your doctor about your ovaries, several factors should be considered:

- **Age:** This is probably the most important factor. Women under 50, or those who have not yet undergone menopause, can continue to benefit significantly from the estrogen their ovaries produce. From preventing bone loss, maintaining cardiovascular health, and supporting brain function estrogen plays an important role in your body. The early loss of estrogen can have significant long-term consequences, which is why age is an initial consideration.

- **Family and personal health history:** Your genetic background plays a significant role in this decision. In the case of having the BRCA, Lynch, or other high-risk genetic mutation, removing your ovaries may be a preventive measure to lower your cancer risk. In these cases, the decision to prevent or reduce your risk of cancer overrides the issues related to hormones, menopause, and other concerns.

- **Hormone replacement therapy:** If you choose to remove your ovaries before natural menopause, you should consider if you are a candidate for Hormone Replacement Therapy (HRT) to manage the symptoms of menopause. HRT, however, can come with its own risks, such as an increased risk of blood clots or high blood pressure, so it's important to weigh these risks and make sure you are a candidate for HRT.

- **Personal preference:** Ultimately, your personal preferences play a huge role in this decision. Many women prefer to keep as many organs intact as possible. As I often hear from my patients, "If the ovaries don't bother me, I'm not going to bother them." This desire to maintain hormonal balance and avoid early menopause is completely understandable. On the other hand, for some women, the potential risk of future ovarian problems—whether from cysts, cancer, or other conditions—may feel like too much of a burden on their peace of mind or quality of life.

Hysterectomy Routes: The Great Escape—Vaginal, Abdominal, or Laparoscopic?

We learned in Chapter 7 about the three major approaches to myomectomy: open abdominal and laparoscopic or robotic. You have the same options for a hysterectomy, as well as a fourth: a vaginal hysterectomy. Let's take a closer look at each of these.

Vaginal Hysterectomy: Finding the Right Candidate

Vaginal hysterectomy can be an excellent option for many women, including those with prolapse, bleeding, or fibroids. It can also be an option for women diagnosed with very early cervical cancer or uterine cancer, as long as there is no evidence that your precancer has spread beyond the cervix to surrounding tissues. The least invasive approach for hysterectomy, vaginal hysterectomy is the preferred approach by the leading Women's Health and surgical organizations. It is considered a total hysterectomy because the surgery is performed through your vagina and the first incision is made around the cervix to loosen the uterus from the vagina. This means the cervix and uterus will both be removed through the vagina. As the name implies, a vaginal hysterectomy typically just involves vaginal surgery which most of the time avoids any abdominal incisions.

The most common reason for a vaginal hysterectomy is uterine prolapse. You may remember that uterine prolapse occurs when the muscles and ligaments of the pelvic floor can no longer support the uterus causing it to slip down into and protrude out of the vagina. During a vaginal hysterectomy your uterus can be removed, and at the same time we can repair the other tissues that are falling down through the vagina. This approach allows you to remove your falling uterus as well as additional issues related to support—all helping to restore function to your pelvic floor.

You may also be a candidate for vaginal hysterectomy to remedy your fibroids if they are small enough to be removed from the vagina. Large fibroids can be challenging and may limit this option. Scar tissue from endometriosis or a prior surgery may also make this approach difficult.

A vaginal approach is possible for people with adenomyosis or abnormal uterine bleeding who have not responded well to medication or more conservative options. In these cases, the bleeding originates from the uterus so a vaginal hysterectomy can be a definitive treatment. For patients with chronic pelvic pain, a vaginal hysterectomy can address symptoms without the need for additional abdominal surgery, which can cause further scarring. A vaginal hysterectomy can be ultimate therapy for chronic pelvic pain as well if other options have failed to provide relief.

Because the vagina is a narrow passage, this can make our ability to visualize all the structures that are necessary during a hysterectomy challenging. We need to ensure that we protect nearby structures like the rectum, bladder, or ureters—the small tubes that bring urine into the bladder. If your surgeon has a concern about removing the uterus through the vagina while keeping the surrounding organs safe, they may recommend an alternative approach.

What Happens During Surgery?

If you and your surgeon both agree that a vaginal hysterectomy is the best approach for you, the procedure follows a generally accepted standard protocol. Vaginal hysterectomies are performed under either general anesthesia (where you are fully asleep), or regional anesthesia like an epidural (where your abdomen and lower part of your body is numbed). After your anesthesia is working, your surgical team will place a catheter in your bladder to drain your urine during the procedure. Your legs are placed in the lithotomy position; in stirrups similar to when you have a Pap smear. If you have lower back issues, it is important to notify your OR team so your back is properly positioned for comfort during the surgery—you may be in this position for a few hours.

In preparation for surgery, your genital area will be cleaned with an antiseptic solution. From here your surgeon will hold your cervix and make an incision in the upper vagina where the cervix, bladder, and vagina meet. The uterus is then carefully separated from the surrounding blood vessels and connective tissue until it is able to be removed. You and your doctor will have already decided whether or not to remove your ovaries and fallopian tubes during this procedure. Occasionally, the fallopian tubes and ovaries may be challenging to remove either because of their location or scar tissue, but in most cases (between 65 to 97.5 percent) both fallopian tubes and ovaries can be removed.

After the uterus is removed, the opening of the vagina, or the vaginal cuff, is typically closed with suture. Some doctors may place a cotton gauze packing in the vagina and your legs are taken out of the lithotomy position, your anesthesia is removed, and you will be transferred to the recovery room for observation.

Recovery and Aftercare

Many patients undergoing a vaginal hysterectomy are discharged the same day, while others may stay in the hospital for a day or two if there are health-related concerns such as bleeding or significant pain. Recovery is relatively swift, with most patients experiencing minimal discomfort due to the procedure's focus on the vaginal area, which is less densely innervated with pain fibers compared to the abdomen.

Typically, it takes about 4 to 6 weeks for the vaginal cuff closure to heal completely. Although the risk of infection is low, we will see you for a follow-up in the office about two weeks after surgery. During this six-week healing period, it's critical to avoid placing anything in your vagina—including tampons, douching, and especially intercourse—to ensure proper healing and minimize complications.

Of all types of hysterectomies, vaginal hysterectomy boasts the shortest recovery time, allowing you to resume your daily activities more quickly. Most importantly, the symptoms that led you to surgery—such as pain, heavy bleeding, or pelvic pressure—will finally be a thing of the past.

Life after a vaginal hysterectomy often feels like a fresh start. With less postoperative discomfort and a quicker recovery process, you'll be back to living fully and freely, enjoying the relief you deserve. Life beyond the symptoms is waiting for you!

Laparoscopic Surgery

After vaginal hysterectomy, laparoscopy is the next best approach for a hysterectomy. You have likely heard of laparoscopic surgery before—more recently rebranded as minimally invasive surgery—it is one of the primary methods gynecologists use to perform abdominal surgeries.

What to Expect

Laparoscopy has evolved significantly over the years and is now a common approach for most gynecological conditions, including fibroids, adenomyosis, and abnormal uterine bleeding that has not responded to other treatments. This approach has also been life-changing for women with endometriosis, who often undergo multiple surgeries to address scarring and inflammation throughout their lifetime. Women with chronic pelvic pain originating from the uterus often find relief through laparoscopic surgery. Similar to a vaginal hysterectomy, laparoscopy may also be used for early-stage cancers of the uterus, cervix, or ovaries.

Laparoscopy is a helpful and minimally invasive approach with several benefits. It's appealing because it offers:

- A faster recovery and return to work time is a common experience for most patients. You should expect to be discharged from the hospital the same day of surgery and feel almost back to baseline in 2 to 4 weeks.
- Generally means little to no hospital admission time and you are discharged to home hours after surgery. No hospital stay may translate to a less expensive surgery.
- Smaller incisions in the skin tend, leading to less trauma on the body, scarring of the skin, and decreased risk for infection when compared to open abdominal surgery.
- Less blood loss and a lower risk of bleeding versus open abdominal surgery.
- Smaller incisions that often translate to less pain during healing and/or use of pain medication, especially narcotics.
- Minimally invasive option for women whose uterus is too large to be removed through the vagina. The uterus can be portioned into smaller pieces and removed from the abdomen without the need for a larger incision.
- Management for patients with a history of pelvic adhesions or scarring while avoiding an open abdominal surgery.
- A good option for patients with prior abdominal surgeries who may have scar tissue and as well as a body that makes a vaginal approach more challenging.

- Low risk of overall complications from laparoscopic surgery.

The downsides:

- There is a risk of injury to the structures inside the body including the intestines, bladder, nerves, and even major blood vessels during surgery.
- If there are any concerns regarding injury, your surgeon may make the decision to make a longer incision on the abdomen and convert to an open abdominal surgery. We do this to better inspect the abdomen and confirm there is no injury to any part of the body. If an injury is found, then we will call in the appropriate specialist to repair the injury.
- There is a risk of infection or incision drainage at any of the several incision sites on the abdomen. While the risk of infection is less than open surgery, it can be most common at the belly button or incision where we remove specimens from the body.
- There is a small risk of hernia—an opening or weakness in the abdominal wall from the incisions placed in the abdomen.

Laparoscopic-Assisted Vaginal Hysterectomy (LAVH)

Laparoscopy can also be combined with vaginal surgery in a procedure known as laparoscopic-assisted vaginal hysterectomy (LAVH). This approach is helpful when the uterus is too high to reach and remove vaginally or for women whose vagina can make visualizing important structures challenging. LAVH can also be considered in patients with a larger uterus or those who have masses on their ovaries. For patients who have a history of abdominal surgery, a combined laparoscopic and vaginal approach can help address scar tissue or other anatomical issues that can make it easier to proceed with the vaginal removal of the uterus.

The Procedure

Laparoscopy is performed under general anesthesia. After your anesthesia has been administered you will be placed in the same lithotomy position as a vaginal hysterectomy. Your abdomen and the vagina are both cleaned with a sterilizing solution and a catheter is placed in your bladder to collect your urine during the surgery. A specialized tool called a uterine manipulator is placed through the cervix and into the uterus. The uterine manipulator helps control the movements of the uterus from the vaginal side to help direct the uterus around the abdomen and then, eventually remove the uterus from the vagina.

Incisions and Trocar Placement

From here your surgeon will make one to three (sometimes four) small incisions on your abdomen, including your belly button. These incisions are used to place trocars (hollow tubes used to pass instruments and a camera into the abdomen) and your abdomen is then filled with carbon dioxide (CO_2) gas that can expand the abdomen so the surgeon can see all of your internal organs and create a space for the surgeon to operate.

As your belly fills with carbon dioxide gas, your body is placed in the Trendelenburg position—where your feet are elevated above your head. This position helps shift your bowel out of your pelvis, into the upper abdomen, which allows for better visualization of your uterus and other pelvic structures.

Visualization and Surgery

Your surgeon will then pass a laparoscope—a thin, lighted tube with a camera on the end—through the trocar which will show the image of your pelvic organs on a television monitor. This setup allows your surgeon to have complete visualization of your abdomen and access to your pelvic structures to complete your hysterectomy.

The uterus is gently moved side to side using the vaginal manipulator to assist in completing your hysterectomy. Once the uterus is detached, it is placed in a surgical bag and either removed from the small incisions in the abdomen or through the vagina. If the uterus is too large to be removed from the vagina, it can be placed into a bag inside your abdomen, sectioned into smaller pieces, and then removed in sections from your abdominal incision. After the uterus is removed, the CO_2 gas is released from your abdomen and your skin is closed (including the vagina if necessary). When your anesthesia is discontinued you will be taken to a postoperative unit to begin your recovery.

Recovery and Aftercare

After your surgery you will wake up in the recovery room. Most patients are discharged home the same day or within twenty-four hours of surgery. If there are any postoperative concerns, you may be admitted to the hospital for observation. The recovery from laparoscopy is often quicker than open abdominal procedures, primarily because the incisions are smaller, distributed across the body, and not concentrated in one central location like with open surgery. You can generally expect a recovery period of about two weeks, but certainly within four weeks, which is shorter than recovery time from an abdominal hysterectomy.

Pain Management

The discomfort after a laparoscopic procedure is usually described as mild to moderate. Most patients find that over-the-counter pain relievers like acetaminophen or ibuprofen work well to relieve discomfort. Occasionally, if needed, you may be prescribed stronger pain medication for the first few days. Unique to laparoscopic procedures is intense (often right shoulder) pain. This is related to residual CO_2 gas that has been trapped in the upper abdomen under the diaphragm, where it causes pressure and irritation to the phrenic nerve, leading to pain in the lower chest and shoulder. This pain can last for a few days, but typically resolves on its own.

The Best of Both Worlds: vNOTES, A New Vaginal Surgery and Laparoscopy Collaboration

The procedure known as vNOTES (vaginal natural orifice transluminal endoscopic surgery) takes the classic vaginal hysterectomy and steps it up a notch with a high-tech laparoscopy. This is an innovative technique that combines the benefits of vaginal surgery and laparoscopy without the need for abdominal incisions. The vNOTES procedure is essentially a method of operating in the abdomen through the vagina. Performed under general anesthesia, it starts with the same positioning and preparation as a vaginal hysterectomy, but here's the upgrade: a small incision is made at the top of the vagina, allowing a special port to access the abdomen. Through this port, a camera and laparoscopic instruments get to work, detaching the uterus and removing it from the vagina. Once the surgery is complete, the incision is closed, the anesthesia is turned off, and you're one step closer to recovery with minimal invasiveness and maximum innovation.

You may be a good candidate if you meet any of the following:

- **Abnormal uterine bleeding:** With or without fibroids.
- **Larger uterus or fibroids:** A uterus that would typically be too big to bring through the vagina with traditional vaginal surgery.
- **Narrow vaginal canal:** Similar to the downside of a vaginal hysterectomy, a narrow vagina can make it hard to see the full scope of the uterus and other body parts surrounding the uterus. This can increase the risk of injury to the structures surrounding the uterus and increase the risk of intestine, bladder, and blood vessel injury.
- **Prior abdominal surgery:** Patients with a history of C-section or abdominal surgeries, which can lead to scar tissue complications can benefit from this approach.
- **Obese patients:** vNOTES can be better suited for heavier patients because it may avoid the anesthesia risk of having to expand the

lungs during laparoscopy. It can also minimize infection risk by avoiding skin incisions on the stomach.

- **Other medical procedures:** Beyond hysterectomy, vNOTES can be used to remove fallopian tubes, ovarian cysts, and fibroids.

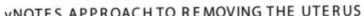

vNOTES APPROACH TO REMOVING THE UTERUS

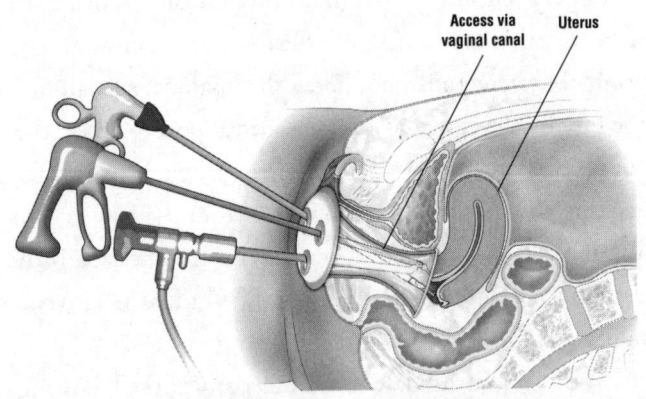

LAPARASCOPIC APPROACH TO REMOVING THE UTERUS

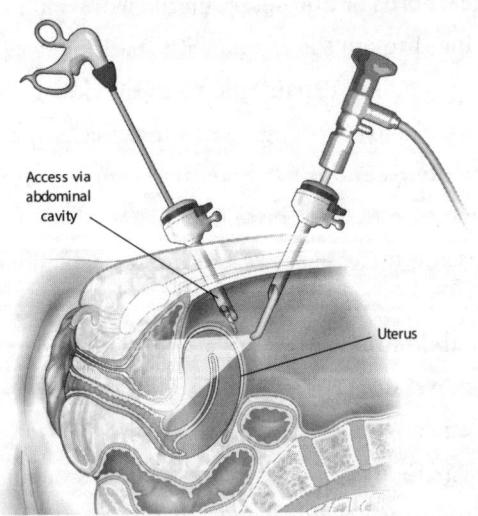

Pros and Cons of vNOTES Hysterectomy vs. Other Methods

Aspect	Vaginal	vNOTES	Laparoscopic	Abdominal
Invasiveness				
	Least	Minimal	Minimal	Most
Scarring				
	No visible scars	No visible scars	Small abdominal scars	Visible abdominal scar
Recovery Time				
	Shorter (4 to 6 weeks)	Shorter (2 to 4 weeks)	Shorter (2 to 4 weeks)	Longer (6 to 8 weeks)
Hospital Stay				
	Home or 1 day	Home or 1 day	Home or 1 day	Longer (2 to 4 days)
Postoperative Pain				
	Less	Less	Moderate	More
Visibility and Precision				
	Limited visibility	Enhanced visibility with laparoscopy	Enhanced visibility with laparoscopy	Most access and significant visibility
Suitability				
	Best for small uterus, prolapse	Suitable for moderate uterine size, benign conditions	Good for most cases, including moderate-size uterus and some adhesions	Suitable for larger uterus, malignancy and patient with prior surgery or significant adhesions
Risks				
	Limited to less complicated cases	Risk of organ injury, requires vNOTES trained surgeon	Risk of organ injury, longer surgical time	Higher risk of infection, longer recovery, can cause adhesions

The vNOTES procedure overcomes the challenges of vaginal surgery, because your surgeon is technically operating in your abdomen. This technique is not limited to hysterectomy, but can be used to remove fallopian tubes, ovarian cysts, and fibroids. It requires special training—which may limit its availability—but this technique is quickly changing gynecology and expanding surgical options for patients.

Recovery

Most patients are discharged home the same day or after a short hospital stay without an abdominal scar. Recovery is the same as with a vaginal hysterectomy, with the average recovery being about 2 to 4 weeks. Some studies suggest that vNOTES patients have less postoperative pain and infection than those having laparoscopic hysterectomies because the abdomen wall and skin are not involved.

Tips for Relieving Shoulder Pain after Laparoscopic Procedure

- *Massage: A gentle massage can help relieve discomfort in the shoulder area.*
- *Walking around: Movement after any surgery is optimal. Walking around can not only help release the trapped gas, movement can also help your intestines return to normal function, and keep you from postoperative complications like blood clots and pneumonia.*
- *Hot or cold packs: You may be given a hot or cold pack in the recovery to help the discomfort. Either is fine and one does not work better than the other.*
- *Over-the-counter pain relievers: Medications like ibuprofen can also help reduce pain and inflammation from the muscles in your shoulder that are irritated from the gas.*

Robotic Hysterectomy

Building on traditional minimally invasive surgeries, robotic surgery has become a popular minimally invasive surgical option. Since 2007 the number of hysterectomies done with robotic surgery has increased dramatically, and today up to 43 percent of laparoscopic hysterectomies use robotic assistance. Despite its name, humans are still very much involved in this surgery, but maybe not in the way you imagine. Robotic surgery uses the same technique as laparoscopy—small incisions in the abdomen to enter and expose your pelvic structures. Unlike laparoscopy, these incisions can be slightly larger, and you may have more incision sites than traditional laparoscopy. A uterine manipulator is also used.

The Procedure

This is where robotic surgery diverges. After the incisions are made on your abdomen, a robotic surgical system is brought close to your body. The robot is "docked" next to your body and its robotic "arms" are attached to the trocars that are inserted into your abdomen. The surgeon moves from the operating table and sits at a console system located in the room. This console provides a 3D, high-definition view of your pelvis offering enhanced visualization of your anatomy. From the console, the surgeon controls the robotic arms which allow for precise and technical surgical movements. Meanwhile a human assistant remains next to your body to help exchange instruments as needed and position the uterus as the surgeon directs. The uterus is removed through the vagina or sectioned into smaller pieces that are then removed from the abdominal incisions.

Most people with fibroids, abnormal bleeding, early gynecological cancers, or endometriosis are suitable candidates for robotic surgery. Robotic surgery is particularly effective in patients who may have complex surgical needs, such as severe pelvic adhesions from previous surgeries, advanced endometriosis with significant scarring, pelvic inflammatory disease, or those with a larger uterus. The small, precise movements of the robot are optimal for managing more complicated anatomy. With laparoscopic or robotic procedures, if there is any suspicion of injury to the bladder, intestines, or excessive bleeding you should be counseled that your procedure can be converted to an open procedure to address any of these issues.

Recovery

Recovery from robotic surgery is similar to recovery from traditional laparoscopy. There may be slightly more discomfort depending on the size and number of abdominal incisions, but most patients can still expect to go home on the same day or after a short hospital stay. The recovery period is generally around 2 to 4 weeks and compared to open surgery patients often experience less pain. The mild or moderate shoulder pain from the CO_2 gas is typically still present and can be managed the same. Similar to laparoscopic procedures, light activity, such as walking, is highly encouraged to prevent complications, but strenuous activities and heavy lifting should be avoided for several weeks based on your doctor's instructions.

Abdominal Hysterectomy

What to Expect

An open or abdominal hysterectomy is the original technique for removing the uterus. It is also the most invasive. An open hysterectomy involves a "bikini" cut (Pfannenstiel incision) that is placed just above where your pubic hair would be. It is the same incision used during a C-section or abdominal myomectomy, but may be shorter or longer based on the size of your uterus. If your uterus is quite large, your surgeon may be compelled to make an incision up and down the middle of your abdomen instead. This is called a vertical midline incision and is often reserved for very large masses or cancer cases to gain much more exposure to the abdomen. The direction of the incision is typically decided in the office with the understanding that it may (but is unlikely) to change after your doctor examines your abdomen in the operating room.

With either incision, with this degree of exposure, we can access all the pelvic and abdominal organs and remove the uterus (possibly tubes and ovaries) in one block. A large uterus is the most common reason for choosing the abdominal approach as it is thought to better visualize blood vessels and surrounding organs, limiting the risk of injury. There is no standard of size of the uterus that should qualify for an open hysterectomy. While studies have shown that a large uterus can be removed laparoscopically, abdominal hysterectomy remains a common route of surgery for uterine fibroids, abnormal uterine bleeding, prolapse, and endometriosis.

Making Use of GnRH Medications

If your doctor is suggesting that you may need a midline incision, please refer to Chapter 6 and reread the section on GnRH medications (Chapter 6). Often a GnRH medication can be used for several months to effectively shrink the uterus and help you avoid a midline incision. This decrease in size may change your incision from an up and down midline to side to side "bikini cut" which is not only more cosmetically appealing but easier to recover from. With time, you may even become a candidate for a laparoscopic or robotic procedure.

The Open Hysterectomy: A Tried-and-True Approach

Your doctor may recommend an open hysterectomy for the following reasons:

- **Size of the uterus:** If you have a large uterus or fibroids that are too large to be removed safely.
- **Pelvic scarring:** Pelvic adhesions due to previous surgery or severe endometriosis can make it challenging to remove the uterus through minimally invasive procedures.

- **Cancer:** Advanced stage uterine, cervical, or ovarian cancer are common reasons for open surgery as the uterus and other organs cannot be sectioned into pieces as it risks spreading cancer.
- **Medical conditions:** Serious lung disease, obesity, and a narrow pelvis or vagina are some reasons that open surgery may be considered as the route may be safer for the surgeon and patient.

An open hysterectomy is always performed under general anesthesia, with you positioned on your back throughout the procedure. Like other surgical approaches, your skin and vagina will be cleaned with a sterilizing solution to minimize the risk of infection. A Foley catheter is placed into your bladder to monitor urine output during and after surgery.

Your surgeon will make either a horizontal "bikini line" incision or a vertical incision on your abdomen. The type and length of the incision depend on factors like the size of your uterus, your body type, and the reason for surgery. For instance, surgeries involving cancer may require a longer incision to sample tissue from other areas of the abdomen.

Once the abdominal layers are opened, the uterus is carefully elevated and separated from its blood supply and surrounding tissues in a systematic manner. After the uterus is removed, the vaginal cuff is closed with sutures. If the cervix is retained, a small internal portion of the cervix is removed to reduce the chance of monthly bleeding or spotting.

After all surgical sites are inspected and no bleeding is noted, the layers of your abdomen are closed. The skin is typically sutured—staples are rarely used—and a bandage is applied to keep the incision clean and dry.

Recovery

This approach offers your surgeon a full-access pass to your entire abdomen, which is particularly important for cases requiring tissue sampling, like cancer surgery. However, this level of access comes with a price: it's more invasive, leading to a longer recovery time and a more noticeable scar. This incision can make getting back to your routine a bit trickier, so be sure to factor it into your recovery timeline and plans. An open hysterectomy is a major surgery with potential risks, but thankfully, the majority of procedures go smoothly. After surgery, you'll head to the recovery room before settling in for a one-to-three-day hospital stay to kick off your recovery journey. While it's a big step, it's often one that paves the way for big relief. Let's break down the aspects you need to consider:

- **Pain management:** This will be a critical part of your postoperative care and you should be prepared for more discomfort than the other surgical options. Your healthcare team should discuss a plan for pain management prior to surgery to ensure comfort and healing. Your pain management options will likely involve stronger medications than the over-the-counter options of laparoscopic or vaginal procedures. As a result of increased discomfort, you will require more days in the hospital as well as an extended period off work— 4 to 6 weeks at least.

- **Infection risk:** With a slightly higher risk of infection, you will need to see your surgeon in two weeks and monitor for infection especially for those patients whose incision is covered by folds of skin. If an infection is suspected, you will receive a course of oral antibiotics to treat the infection. Rarely is more than an oral antibiotic needed. It is important to keep the incision clean and dry. Special lotions, soaps, or astringents are not needed during this time.

- **Blood loss:** With an open hysterectomy, there is a possibility of slightly more blood loss. You should have your blood levels monitored the day(s) after surgery. If the blood loss in surgery was more than expected, oral and IV iron, or even a blood transfusion may be part of your recovery.

* * *

As you can see, understanding your surgical options for hysterectomy is crucial to knowing what the best approach is for you. Now, your goal is to center your health needs in the context of your surgical options. This is where your understanding of your body, personal values, and collaboration with your doctor intersect to make the right decision for you. Remember that this decision is not about loss, but about reclaiming your health and well-being. You have deeply thought about this decision and are ready for bold action. With thoughtful preparation and partnership with your healthcare team, you are ready to prepare for the preoperative process and launch your healthcare journey into full speed.

PART THREE

If You Opt to Have a Hysterectomy

10

❦

The Pre-Op Prep Talk

Powering Up for Your Hysterectomy

S
o, we are finally here. You have said the words, "I am ready for my hysterectomy" and you want to move forward. You have tried it all—multiple prescriptions, procedures, and diets. Or maybe you are at your breaking point with the many doctor visits, ER visits, blood transfusions, and countless days where you have missed out on life. Maybe you've resisted this decision because it is so heavy with emotion. If you're anything like my patients, I know you've experienced a range of emotions from anger to fear to maybe even sadness. Anger for having to deal with these issues in the first place. Fear in knowing that surgery is a big deal and not knowing what the next steps may be. And sadness as you perhaps mourn the loss of part of yourself that is so precious to you. All of these emotions and more are very appropriate. Despite this, you know that it is time. You have come to this decision because you have not been living life to its fullest. It is your body, and you are ready to regain control. It is time to reclaim your life from years of pain and bleeding.

First let me congratulate you on reaching this decision. I have had so many patients express relief and peace after making this decision. I've found that this is even more true after they have had their surgery and are fully healed. Can you imagine how good you'll feel when you know your life is no longer held hostage by the threat of your uterus?

Even though you have reached a point of decision-making, there is still so much to consider. What will happen, and how? You are rightfully worried about pain, surgery complications, and life after a hysterectomy. I've got you; this chapter is your pre-op pep talk. Most importantly, you should come out of this chapter feeling confident in the knowledge of all the steps that will happen before your surgery, and how you can discuss them with your care team.

Selecting Your Surgeon

First things first: your surgeon should be one you trust and feel comfortable talking through your concerns with. If you've been with your gynecologist for several years now, love them, and feel that they have expertly guided you through the process of coming to this decision, you're in the most ideal situation. When a doctor and patient have a good working relationship and there is trust and mutual respect it is both empowering and comforting to move forward with the plan you have discussed together.

However, if you are not in that situation, it is time to change it. My grandmother used to say, *A closed mouth doesn't get fed*. I didn't understand her Southern wisdom until I got older but now, I get it: you won't find help unless you ask for help. This is true for your surgeon, too. Talk to your friends, family, and coworkers about your need for a good gynecologist. Folks who have a good experience will be happy to refer you and tell you all about their experience. Even if they didn't have a hysterectomy with this doctor, their enthusiasm can still be valuable.

Listen for comments like: "she listens," "she's so good," "I felt so cared for," "I don't even mind going to her office," and "I trust her." While surgical skills are important, the doctor-patient relationship is also important, right? A referral from a trusted friend or family member can be an important resource to finding your "person" for this journey.

When you meet your possible doctor, your Spidey sense will click in. Trust this instinct. Pay attention to how they listen, ask meaningful questions, and answer your questions in plain, accessible language. These are signs that you may have found a potential good fit.

You can also cast a really wide net by searching on your insurance provider's website. The home page typically has a "find a doctor" tab that will allow you to search by area, gender, and specialty. Look for physicians in your area that may take your insurance. When you find someone who piques your interest, read their bylines to find out if they perform surgery themselves or have any other specific practice interests, like fibroids or endometriosis. Another option is to visit the website of a hospital you trust. This may ensure that your doctor operates out of a hospital that you are familiar with and has a good reputation in the community for trusted care and good outcomes.

You can also ask your primary care doctor—actually you can ask all your other doctors, including your internal medicine doctor, dentist, or anyone who cares for you may have a recommendation. Honey, let me tell you. Doctors talk, especially to each other. We know the inside scoop on who we trust for a particular procedure. Your PCP can be your medical inside (wo)man to all the local favorite gynecologists in your community. Your personal doctors can be invaluable in helping you sift through well-respected community doctors. Many of them may work closely with a preferred group of gynecologists and can recommend someone who might be a great fit for your needs. This does not mean that you have to willingly go with their recommendation, but it is a good start to perhaps narrow your search to find the doctor that is right for you.

If you choose a doctor who stops feeling like a good fit for you at any point in the process, it is okay to switch it up. I know too many women who stay stuck with the wrong person because they feel bad about leaving or think they're not allowed to change their minds. Let me tell you: you can change your mind at any point. If you don't feel heard, or you feel rushed or frustrated or are having doubts, I encourage you to bring this up with your doctor, but if this is not your personality or does not change you may consider starting your search again.

The Preoperative Process

Once you've found your doctor and have established a relationship with them, it is time to get down to business. There are several factors that you and your doctor will need to consider to help create a solid plan for your surgery. This process can differ from office to office and across the hospital system, but the point is that there are some boxes that need to be checked before you can move forward with surgery. For me, the first thing I recommend is to choose a date.

Choose a Day

Not every office is the same, but I encourage patients to pick their surgical day as the first step of your pre-op process. With this set, we can then work backward to address any medical, insurance, or other issue that may pop up before the surgery. After you have chosen a day, your doctor's office will contact the hospital to provide your details to reserve a time slot for your procedure. The office will also start the authorization process with your insurance company, which usually starts with the first question: What day is the surgery?

Most of the time the authorization process with your insurance company is straightforward, but occasionally there can be some roadblocks. Your doctor's office is typically responsible for this and does not involve you. After you have chosen your surgical day, your doctor's office should also schedule a postoperative exam check two weeks after your surgery, to make sure you're recovering to plan.

Pre-op Examinations

As part of the early visits to your surgeon's office, we want to conduct a thorough examination of you, including your vital signs—weight, blood pressure, heart rate, and temperature, as well as take a detailed medical history. This is not the time to withhold any significant medical history and medications you are taking no matter how insignificant or embarrassing. For example, last year I operated on a patient who had prior abdominoplasty or "tummy tuck." She mentioned that her surgery was performed in the United States, but when I started her surgery, there were telltale signs that her surgery was done outside of this country.

Why does this matter? The omission of this detail not only made her surgery longer, it was also more complicated and made the surgery potentially life-threatening. If I had this information up-front, her preoperative counseling and even surgical approach would have been different. So, it's important to be up front and provide accurate and complete information as it can impact your health and the success of your surgery.

Next steps include an exam, which usually involves two to three parts. The first is simply the placement of our hands on your abdomen to better understand the size and shape of your uterus. Along with imaging, this helps us understand the general size, shape, and mobility of your uterus. Mobility refers to how easily your uterus can be manipulated or moved around in your body. This helps inform which surgical approach may be best. For example, if you have a uterus that is hard to move around or completely immobile, it may suggest concerns like scar tissue and endometriosis, which can influence the placement of incision or the type of surgery we recommend.

The second phase is typically a pelvic exam. With your consent, a pelvic exam starts just by looking at your vulva and we may ask you to cough or bear down. Several hearty coughs help us assess the strength of your pelvic floor. After this general observation, we then proceed to an internal physical exam. During the internal exam, one or two lubricated gloved fingers are placed in the vagina while the other hand is pressed down on your abdomen. This gives us more information about mobility, the size, position, and shape of your uterus and ovaries as well as any potential scarring from prior surgery, endometriosis, or infection.

Finally, you may need to prepare for a rectal exam. I know they can be uncomfortable but in some cases they can be very useful for offering information about mobility, and for people with endometriosis it can help us understand the extent of possible scarring from endometriosis in the back of your uterus which can impact the approach of the surgery. Your doctor should ask your consent before performing a rectal exam so it's not a surprise.

If you are over forty or have a family history of breast cancer, your doctor may request an up-to-date mammogram and/or a recent breast exam. If a mass is noted or your mammogram is abnormal, this will take precedence over your hysterectomy. For similar reasons, you will need a recent Pap smear, which will test for cervical cancer and presence of the human papillomavirus (HPV). If you have either an abnormal Pap smear or a current HPV infection, your doctor is going to want to follow the appropriate recommendations to ensure that you have no signs of early cancer. This would significantly alter the counseling and approach to your hysterectomy.

We also test for vaginal infections such as gonorrhea, chlamydia, trichomoniasis or bacterial vaginosis before surgery. Though this is not always necessary, these infections can complicate your healing process so know that your doctor may recommend testing as a precaution. Of these, bacterial vaginosis is known to cause infection at the vaginal cuff—the top of the vagina that is sewn together after the cervix is removed. Bacterial vaginosis is highly associated with an increased risk of vaginal cuff infections following a hysterectomy. Fortunately, all of these infections however are easily treated with oral antibiotics and should be treated before surgery.

Pre-op Doctor's Appointment

After your evaluation with your gynecologist, you'll be sent to a preoperative appointment with your family medicine or internal medicine doctor. This preoperative examination, often referred to as the pre-op exam, may be the most important evaluation before your surgery—it is essentially the gatekeeper to your surgery. Not only will your hospital require this evaluation, it is our formal way of ensuring your overall health has been evaluated, optimized as much as possible and you can move forward with this intermediate risk surgery.

The pre-op exam does not simply "clear" you for surgery nor does it guarantee that you will not have any intraoperative or postoperative complications. It is a comprehensive evaluation of almost every system of your body and—if necessary—recommendations to implement to optimize your health for what is considered an intermediate risk surgery. This visit and subsequent recommendations can help decrease the length of your hospital stay and the chance that your surgery is postponed or canceled. To have a productive consultation, you need to tell your doctor what type of hysterectomy you are having so you should disclose if the plan is for an open, laparoscopic, or vaginal procedure. The surgical approach may influence recommendations related to new or chronic medical conditions you have. Your consultation will also include recommendations and a plan for preoperative blood work and testing. It will conclude with interventions that can minimize your risk for complications.

Surgical complications generally fall into one of three categories: infectious, respiratory, and cardiac, in that order. While cardiac complications are least common, understandably they can have the greatest impact on your health. This is why the first priority is an evaluation of your heart, typically starting with an EKG. This quick, painless, and inexpensive test evaluates the electrical signals moving through your heart. It makes sure the signals are regular and warns of an irregular heartbeat. A normal EKG typically signals that your heart can manage the stress of surgery and anesthesia. If you are forty or older or have high blood pressure, heart disease, diabetes, or really any chronic medical condition you should expect to have an EKG. Even if you are perfectly healthy, an EKG is standard before surgery. If the EKG is abnormal then additional testing is required, most often an echocardiogram, or echo for short. An echo is an ultrasound of the heart that helps us analyze the movement of the valves and walls of the heart. You also may be asked to have a cardiac stress test, which involves walking on a treadmill or receiving IV medication if you cannot walk to assess your heart's ability to respond to stress. If you require either an echo or cardiac stress test it is very likely that your primary care doctor will recommend you consult with a cardiologist prior to proceeding with surgery.

Your medical doctor will listen to your lungs to ensure they are clear and that you have no cough or congestion that could incite respiratory complications. It is unlikely you will need a chest X-ray if you do not have chronic lung disease, but it may be necessary if you have an unexplained new cough or shortness of breath. Chronic lung disease like asthma or chronic obstructive pulmonary disease (COPD) may require a pulmonary function testing prior to surgery. Additionally, we assess your lungs' ability to exchange oxygen by measuring your oxygen saturation with a pulse oximeter—a small monitor placed most often on your finger when the office collects your vital signs. At rest this number should be above 95 percent and anything less may be considered abnormal and warrant an evaluation especially if lung disease is present.

Asthma is a common, chronic lung condition. If you have asthma, it is crucial for it to be well controlled in the weeks to months leading up to your surgery. Asthmatics have a higher risk of airway spasm, losing oxygen saturation, coughing, excessive secretions, and pneumonia after anesthesia. In this group, pulmonary functions tests (PFTs) may be very important. You also may be prescribed oral and inhaled steroids before and after surgery, which will help prevent and reduce the inflammation and constriction of the airways that may happen when the breathing tube is placed (intubation) during general anesthesia. Your anesthesiologist will likely have you use your inhaler just prior to entering the operating room. Your inhaler will then follow you for use in the recovery room and beyond as it is important to manage your respiratory health before and after the surgical procedure.

Your family doctor will also do a smoking assessment. Whether you smoke tobacco, marijuana, or vape, smoking will have one of the greatest negative impacts on your surgery and recovery. Tobacco smokers, in particular, have a significantly higher risk of postoperative complications compared to nonsmokers. During and after surgery your body enters "trauma recovery mode," knowing it has to heal itself and fight infection. This is when your body's need for oxygen is at an all-time high, and smoking thwarts this process. Smoking damages the cells' ability to clear mucus, which impairs oxygen exchange and increases your risk for infection and other respiratory complications.

Smoking can impair healing of your incision and increase your risk for infection. Smoking slows the delivery of healing oxygen and delays healing signals that the body needs to make the collagen needed to heal. The chemical stress and toxins in smoke also slow down cells designed to fight infection, leading to more surgical site infections. If you are a smoker, you will be asked to quit smoking for at least eight weeks before surgery. This will give time for the cells that clear the mucus to recover and allow for better oxygen exchange.

After surgery, we encourage all patients to perform deep breathing exercises to reduce your risk of lung infection. This is especially important for people with lung disease and smokers. For these exercises, you will receive an incentive spirometer, a handheld device that measures the volume of the air inhaled into the lungs. When you breathe deeply it gives you immediate visual feedback on how deeply (or not) you are breathing. Your care team will give you instruction on how to use this device to properly open up your lungs, cough up phlegm, and reduce the risk of lung infections like pneumonia. Plan on using your incentive spirometer to take a minimum of at least ten deep breaths every hour you are awake, especially if you are overweight or having open abdominal surgery.

Your doctor will also review your medication list and advise you which meds you should hold before surgery. Popular weight-loss medications, blood thinners, and nonsteroidal anti-inflammatory drugs (like ibuprofen or aspirin) should be discontinued or held off prior to surgery. Certain vitamins or herbal medications that may cause bleeding such as aloe, ginger, ginkgo, garlic, green tea, grapefruit, ginseng, oregano, or vitamin E should also be stopped before surgery. Your PCP will tell you when you can restart these and other medications.

At the end of this evaluation, your PCP will complete paperwork detailing their suggestions to optimize your health for this intermediate risk procedure. This report will be sent to your gynecologist's office for reference on the day of surgery and will be added to your hospital chart.

Blood Work

As part of your evaluation, certain preoperative blood work will be collected. Current recommendations suggest tailoring labs to the individual so you may or may not need everything reviewed here. Also, remember not to stress if a lab returns abnormal—this occasionally happens. It does not always mean your surgery will be canceled. You and your medical team typically have time to repeat or optimize the lab value before a major surgery. You can expect your team to run the following tests:

- **Complete blood count (CBC):** Iron deficiency anemia (IDA) is a common blood condition where the levels of iron or red blood cells that carry iron are low. Iron deficiency anemia is the most common cause of anemia worldwide. Even though IDA is common, it is still a concern because it puts stress on your heart and brain. It is the strongest predictor for the need of a blood transfusion during or after surgery. Upward of 22 percent of women preparing for hysterectomy or myomectomy are anemic. Since most patients are eager to avoid a blood transfusion, if we find that you are anemic prior to surgery, you will likely be referred to a hematologist, a doctor that specializes in conditions of the blood, for further management. The CBC, or complete blood count, is a key test to assess IDA and your blood's iron levels. The CBC test offers several ways to analyze your iron stores, but most importantly we look at values called the hemoglobin and hematocrit. Hemoglobin represents the protein that carries oxygen from your lungs and delivers it to the rest of your body; it is the reason your blood is red. The CBC also offers another marker of iron level—the hematocrit. The hematocrit reveals what percentage of your blood is made up of red blood cells versus other cells. If either the protein that carries oxygen is low (hemoglobin) or if the number of red blood cells is low (hematocrit) you may be considered anemic.

Lab values that determine anemia can change from laboratory to laboratory but in general if your results fall below the laboratory standard you will be considered anemic. Hemoglobin values for females is 12 to 16 g/dl and normal hematocrit levels range from 36 to 48 percent. If your results are lower than these values your surgery may need to be postponed until they have increased to a safe range. Iron supplementation (either with diet or oral supplements) is the main way we can increase iron stores. Adjusting your diet to include more iron-rich animal or plant-based foods and/or oral pills can boost your levels in a few weeks. With the help of a hematologist, you can raise your iron quickly with intravenous (IV) iron. Many studies have noted that IV iron is more effective and better tolerated than oral iron. IV iron can deliver a large amount of iron for your body to incorporate into your red blood cells. You can receive anywhere from one to four weekly IV transfusions, each taking about fifteen to thirty minutes. During this time, you may receive about 1,000 mg of iron versus the typical 325 mg (65 mg) in an oral supplement. Your transfusions can be timed to peak your iron stores just in time for surgery. Your signs of anemia (fatigue, weakness, et cetera) may improve as soon as several days after your first transfusion. In a matter of weeks to two months, your iron levels can increase, and you may proceed safely to surgery. Intravenous iron may be new to you, but consider it a valuable option to treat significant anemia or if you cannot tolerate oral medications. In my experience, the benefits of iron transfusions far outweigh the risks, allowing you to address your iron deficiency quickly and proceed to surgery as planned.

- **Comprehensive metabolic panel (CMP):** This test will assess your liver and kidneys, which are crucial for processing of medications and anesthesia. It ensures these organs can handle the stress of surgery and anesthesia.

- **Prothrombin time (PT), partial thromboplastin time (PTT):** These are tests that check how long it takes your blood to clot. They are usually ordered if you are on blood thinners, have a family or personal history of a bleeding disorder, or have evidence of liver disease.

- **Thyroid-stimulating hormone (TSH):** You may not be screened for thyroid disease if you do not have anything in your history that suggests thyroid disease. If you have thyroid disease and are on thyroid medication, you should monitor your thyroid annually. If you have normal labs within the last three to six months and your medication is stable, then you should be able to proceed with surgery.

- **Urinalysis or urine culture:** If you have a history of urinary tract infections (UTIs) this will ensure you do not have an infection before you enter surgery. Otherwise, this test is not required.

- **Urine pregnancy test:** You would be surprised how often people discover they are pregnant on the day of the surgery. Because it is such a frequent occurrence, a urine pregnancy test is always done preoperatively and especially on the day of surgery in all reproductive-age women. Sometimes postmenopausal women will even be asked to take a pregnancy test. What can I say, unexpected pregnancies can happen, and it is imperative that we confirm you are not pregnant before surgery. Needless to say, if you are pregnant before surgery your procedure will be rescheduled or canceled.

- **Hemoglobin A1C:** This test is an important marker for diabetics. If you are over forty-five, have diabetes, or risk factors for diabetes your doctor may check this number. For diabetics, strict sugar control is crucial for optimal healing and to minimize infection.

A Note about Obesity

If your body mass index (BMI) is over 30kg/m², you may be classified as obese—but let's be real: BMI is just a piece of the puzzle when it comes to a measure of someone's health. While the medical field is (thankfully) moving away from using BMI as the sole indication of your fitness for surgery, years of research and clinical experience have shown that heavier patients may face unique challenges when it comes to anesthesia and surgery.

Your surgeon and anesthesiologist should review these risks with you, but I wanted to make sure you feel informed and empowered in this process. If weight is a potential surgical risk for you, the key is to identify those risks early and put strategies in place to minimize your risk of complications both during and after surgery.

Anesthesia-Related Risks

Surgical procedures with anesthesia can pose more complications for patients classified as obese or overweight, including:

- **IV line placement issues:**
  - Finding and securing an intravenous line can be more challenging. Veins can be harder to locate and access due to increased soft tissue thickness. This can make finding a suitable vein for the IV line more time-consuming and slightly complicated. Occasionally, your anesthesiologist may use an ultrasound machine, commonly called a "vein finder" to help locate a suitable vein to administer fluids and other medications.

- Dehydration or low blood pressure can further complicate vein visibility and accessibility. Make sure you are intentional about hydration in the days leading into surgery to help your veins achieve maximum visibility.

- If you are a notoriously "hard stick," then please consider using your hand for the initial IV access. As more fluids are administered (especially if you are dehydrated), larger veins and more comfortable veins in your arm will eventually show up to the party.

- Occasionally, the placement of a central venous catheter (a larger IV line into a vein in the neck or chest) may be suggested if arm, hand, or even foot veins are not accessible for your procedure.

- **Airway management:**
  - Depending on how your weight is distributed, obesity can lead to excess tissue around the neck and throat. When you are on your back (as is the case in surgery), the weight of your neck tissue can obstruct or block your airway. This may mean that for even short procedures, your anesthesiologist should be prepared for several airway options and may recommend intubation (inserting a thin tube into your airway) to keep your airway open and make it easier to provide oxygen to your lungs.

  - Your PCP and anesthesiologist will also ask you about symptoms related to sleep apnea. If you have sleep apnea—a sleep disorder that causes breathing to repeatedly stop or become shallow during sleep—this can increase your risk for airway complications. Conditions like obstructive sleep apnea (common in obese patients) add to the complexity by increasing the challenge of keeping your airway open during anesthesia.

  - A larger tongue or narrow airway can make inserting a breathing tube more difficult. The anesthesiologist will then likely use a small camera to direct the breathing tube past your tongue and securely into your airway.

- **Lung expansion challenges:**
  - During surgery, excess weight, particularly on the chest and abdomen, can compress the lungs. This can become even more challenging during laparoscopy and even when lying flat for a prolonged time. Your team will consider anesthesia adjustments to maintain oxygen levels, including giving oxygen before and during surgery. Position changes during surgery may also be necessary to improve your lungs ability to move air and keep oxygen levels in a normal range.
  - After surgery, the use of an incentive spirometer (a breathing exercise device) several times an hour is important to encourage deep breathing and lung expansion. We are also going to encourage you to move your body several times a day. Standing upright will help you move air into the deepest part of your lungs and minimize risk for pneumonia.

Now let's review some of the surgical risks that may come up due to increased weight. These are issues your team will guide you through and prepare for to minimize the risk of complication:

- **Increased blood loss:** Increased soft tissue can make surgery more difficult and longer-essentially more time for bleeding. Larger blood vessels and vascular networks can mean more bleeding during incisions and dissection. To minimize bleeding your surgeon and surgical team are going to be intentional about using advanced techniques to minimize your blood loss. This can range from medications before and during surgery, the types of instruments we use during surgery, and reducing the overall time spent operating. A blood transfusion will be prepared and available in the event it is needed.

- **Higher risk of infection:** You may receive a higher dose of antibiotic that has been adjusted to your weight before the procedure begins. We will also sterilize your skin before the procedure, but it is critical that you keep the skin clean and dry as it heals. You should look for and report any signs of early infection so your team can start treatment early before an infection can spread. The reasons risks of infection increases are:
    - There is less blood flow to fatty tissue which slows down healing and delivery of immune cells to the surgical site—which can impair wound healing.
    - Increased moisture and warmth on the skin are a lovely home for bacteria and raise the risk of surgical site infections.
    - Obesity related conditions like diabetes also compromise your ability to heal and make you more susceptible to infection.
- **Blood clots:** A blood clot is a very serious event and can be life threatening. Being overweight or obese puts pressure on the veins and slows the blood in the venous system making it more likely to develop blood clots. Sluggish blood flow combined with the limited mobility after surgery is the perfect storm for a blood clot. We try to minimize the risk of blood clots by asking you to move as soon as early as you can after surgery. We will also place compression stockings or use sequential compression devices (SCDs) to encourage blood circulation in the legs. In cases where the risk of a blood clot is significant, you may also receive blood thinning shots before and after surgery to prevent blood clots.

Understanding these risks isn't meant to alarm you, but to prepare and empower. With proper precautions and personalized surgical planning, these risks can be significantly reduced. Discuss your concerns with your surgeon and anesthesiologist to ensure a plan is in place to manage these challenges effectively. A collaborative, proactive approach is key to a safe and successful procedure.

Informed Consent Visit

About 1 to 2 weeks before surgery, I schedule patients for a follow-up visit which I prefer to call an informed consent visit. It's a mix of business and education. We make sure that your preoperative evaluation by your medical doctor is complete and received by the office. We are looking to ensure your blood work results are normal, an EKG or any other testing is complete and normal, as well as your medical history is complete and documented on forms that will be forwarded to the hospital. If anything is missing, this serves as a gentle nudge to move things along.

The focus, however, is on you. Together we will confirm the type of surgery we have agreed to and once again review the known risks and benefits of surgery. From my experience, these concerns are best discussed prior to surgery and not on the day of surgery when you are already full of emotion and could potentially send your blood pressure skyrocketing.

This visit allows us to address your specific questions and concerns about surgery. Most times one visit is enough, but sometimes two are required. Given the limited time doctors often get to spend with patients, it is best that we have more time to manage the information in smaller, more digestible pieces, rather than feel overwhelmed. These visits can carry a lot of information, so it is a good idea to come prepared to take notes.

The foundation of surgical consent is first that you have a clear understanding of what your diagnosis is and why you are having surgery. In this case, it may be that you have endometriosis, fibroids, pelvic pain, pelvic organ prolapse, or a combination of these. I will explain the reasonable risks and benefits of surgery. Informed consent also means understanding your alternative options, including the option to do nothing about your condition. Finally, informed consent means you understand the important information we have discussed and are not coerced to proceed with surgery.

We will also talk about your realistic expectations and goals for after surgery. If you have a prolapse, is your goal to be able to exercise without feeling pressure or are you more concerned about urinary symptoms? If you have endometriosis, is your goal to have pain-free intercourse or to stop having periods all together. It is important that we both understand your expectations, the reality of surgery, and a reasonable timeline to reach those goals.

We will also reaffirm your decision to proceed with surgery and document our conversation of your understanding of the risk, benefits, and alternatives in your medical record. Although it is not common, when it is thought to be appropriate surgeons and patients may coordinate to combine multiple surgical procedures at the same time. For example, an abdominoplasty, commonly known as a tummy tuck, might be scheduled with your hysterectomy. We often call this as a "hyst 'n' tuck"— meaning after your gynecologist addresses your planned hysterectomy a plastic surgeon will remove excessive skin and fat to optimize your time spent under anesthesia. Combined surgeries are not limited to a tummy tuck, but may also include removing your gallbladder, breast surgery, or other procedures. To confirm you are properly consented for all of your surgeries, each surgeon should complete a separate and detailed informed consent with you. In addition to consents that permit surgery, there are also separate consents that document which interventions or treatment(s) you decline or refuse. This is most commonly a discussion and practice for patients who refuse blood transfusion, any blood products, or older patients who may decline forms of life support.

The Fine Print: What Your Surgeon Needs You to Know
Every surgery has inherent risks. Your doctor will discuss these risks with you as well as what you can do to minimize them.

Infection
The first thing I review with patients is the risk of infection. Your skin, a specialized organ, plays a key role in preventing infection and is home to about 1.5 trillion bacteria. While most bacteria are harmless or even

beneficial, some of the one thousand species of bacteria on our skin can cause injury, such as during surgery. Once the skin is cut, bacteria can quickly enter your tissue and blood and may lead to infection. The risk of an infection is lowest with vaginal hysterectomy (.9 percent) and highest with abdominal hysterectomy (1.7 percent). Fortunately, your risk of infection is low due to many preventive measures in place to reduce the risk of infection and promote healing.

To prevent infections, it is important to prepare the skin for surgery. Some surgeons may ask you to bathe the night before with a special chlorhexidine solution or antimicrobial soap. Similar to the night before washing, some surgeons may ask you to remove body hair. Hair removal is controversial. While removing hair can help when closing the skin or applying the dressing, some studies claim that certain types of hair removal can cause skin infections. The general consensus is that there's no real difference in infection if you remove hair or not. However, if you are asked to remove some hair, using clippers and depilatory cream are preferred over razors, and hair should be removed the day before or the day of surgery.

Metal jewelry should be removed before surgery because it can conduct electric current and pose a risk of causing burns on your skin. Nose and/or oral jewelry should definitely be removed because it can interfere with anesthesia and also pose a burn risk. Navel rings can either be removed the day before or you can place a plastic spacer in the piercing until after the surgery is over. You can replace the navel ring five to ten days later. Just remember to disinfect and clean the skin before reinserting the metal back into the piercing.

To help further reduce your risk of infection, do not plan any new tattoos before surgery. Your skin is a protective barrier, and fresh tattoos offer the opportunity for bacteria to enter and infect the skin. You should avoid any tattoos, including microblading, for at least 2 to 6 weeks before surgery. If an incision needs to cross a previous tattoo site, it can't be helped. We will do our best to minimize any disruption, but you can always revisit your tattoo artist or plastic surgeon if any irregularity or scarring is a concern.

Antibiotics are another line of defense against infection. For an abdominal hysterectomy you will receive at least one universal antibiotic. These antibiotics are chosen because they cover bacteria found on the skin, abdomen, and vagina. Antibiotics are selected with best practices in mind, allergies, your weight, and the consideration of bacterial resistance in your local area. They are given in your IV within sixty minutes of the skin incision and periodically re-dosed if required. You will be given antibiotics postoperatively if you develop an infection.

As part of infection prevention, your skin will also be cleaned with an alcohol-based solution, unless you have a known allergy to it. The vagina is also cleaned with a special solution (chlorhexidine gluconate or povidone iodine) to reduce the risk of bacteria moving from the vagina into the abdomen or the vaginal cuff. If you have a known sensitivity to iodine or chlorhexidine, we use alternatives like sterile water and baby shampoo. Let your surgeon know if you have any reaction or sensitivity to these solutions after surgery.

During surgery, your anesthesiologist will keep you warm with a special gown or blanket that blows warm air over your upper body throughout the surgery. Even slight deviations in your body temperature can stimulate your body's stress response and can lead to a two-to-three-fold increase in wound infection, increase blood loss, and cause significant physical discomfort.

In the operating room we maintain strict protocols to minimize your risk of infection. This can range from tight control of your blood sugar, limiting the traffic in and out of the operating room, and minimizing blood loss which reduces your risk for transfusions. When your procedure is complete, we will then put on all new sterile gloves, gowns, and surgical instruments to close your skin to make sure no possible bacteria from the first part of the surgery contaminates the last part of the surgery. Rarely, you may have a small tube called a surgical drain placed in your lower abdomen. Drains help remove fluid from the body and can help alert us of a potential complication. While rarely used, a drain can be a source of infection, so we aim to remove them as soon as it is medically appropriate. Your bladder catheter, another type of drain, is typically removed either immediately after surgery or within twenty-four hours to reduce the risk of a bladder infection.

"All Indicated Procedures"

Your doctor may use the phrase "all indicated procedures" when discussing the risks of surgery. This means that—in the event of an unlikely complication—you are giving us your permission to take care of the complication. Basically, it means if there is an injury to any part of your body, we have your consent to repair the concern even if it means another procedure or the consultation of other specialists. It does not mean we can choose to perform unrelated surgery, like removing a mole, but if the bladder or intestines are injured, you give consent to repair the injury according to the standard of care.

The risk for unplanned surgery is unlikely but may be slightly increased if this is not your first abdominal surgery. Why? After each abdominal surgery—especially C-sections and myomectomies—you can form fibrous bands of tissue or scar known as adhesions between your uterus and other organs. If you have had an infection such as pelvic inflammatory disease or have endometriosis, we know that inflammation and scar tissue are a part of these conditions. Infection, endometriosis, or prior surgery all can cause scar tissue to form between the organs making them stick together when they should glide smoothly over each other. In these situations, delicate structures like the bladder, intestines, and blood vessels can be injured and must be repaired. Every surgeon, including myself, has experienced an unexpected injury to the bladder, intestines, or blood vessel. It is not a sign of a bad procedure, but a known risk of any surgery. These injuries are never intentional. For your health, recovery, and safety the most important issue is that the injury was recognized, repaired while in the operating room, and explained to you after surgery.

Bleeding and Risk of Blood Transfusion

The uterus has several sources of blood flow and can bleed quickly if any of these vessels are not secured. To manage the risk of blood-related complications we focus on optimizing your blood levels before the OR and minimizing blood loss during your procedure. Closer to surgery, we will reassess you for anemia, especially if you suffer from heavy periods. If you are low or borderline, we have options to help reduce anemia. One option is to consider medications that can reduce bleeding such as oral contraceptive medication, antifibrinolytics, GnRH agonists, or a hormonal IUD. Even a minor intervention like a Dilation and Curettage or a Uterine Artery Embolization can help. The goal is to lighten your periods and preserve your blood volume leading up to surgery.

The second is to conserve blood loss with a thoughtful surgical plan. One device that may be available in your hospital is called the cell saver, which is a cool name for a machine that does exactly what it sounds like—save your red blood cells. This machine suctions blood lost during surgery, stores it in a sterile container, and after the surgery will rinse, clean, and return the blood to your circulation. It is very much like a self-transfusion. At the end of the surgery up to 80 percent of the blood lost in surgery can be returned to you. If there is not enough blood to return, this is actually a good sign that minimal blood was lost. For individuals looking to avoid transfusion for personal or religious reasons, a cell saver is a great option to help blood loss during surgery.

While not commonly used for otherwise healthy patients, erythropoietin (EPO) is a medication that can boost red blood cell production and increase your hemoglobin levels. It is a once-weekly injection about three weeks before an elective procedure together with IV iron. EPO does not substitute for iron supplementation but is used as a complement to iron as a part of some anemia treatment plans. EPO is used in multiple settings including patients with cancer, chronic kidney disease, significant anemia, or those who cannot receive blood for personal and religious reasons. Generally, the decision to use EPO is influenced by your ability to increase your iron levels, urgency of the surgery, your healthcare team, and the need to avoid blood transfusion. Risks with EPO are rare but can include high blood pressure and the small risk of blood clot.

Your surgeon will use meticulous surgical techniques to help reduce blood loss during surgery. In addition, to our surgical technique we may use various locally applied treatments called hemostatic agents to stop bleeding. These agents use your body's clotting mechanisms to form clots and slow bleeding; they can be liquid, foam, or fiber-like products that activate local blood clotting mechanisms and stop bleeding.

Other interventions to minimize bleeding include surgical instruments that seal blood vessels. During your surgery, your anesthesiologist will work to manage your blood pressure, IV fluids, and body temperature to help minimize bleeding. Post-surgery we will also aim to limit the number of blood draws to reduce further contributing to anemia. Using smaller collection tubes alongside less frequent blood draws we can help minimize the chance you become anemic by just being in the hospital.

Many patients ask, "Why can't I just donate my own blood?" Donating your own blood, also known as autologous transfusion or preoperative autologous donation (PAD), makes sense. I understand your thinking—if you are not anemic and facing surgery, why not store some of your own blood for transfusion during or after surgery. The data, however, suggests that PAD may not be as helpful as you might think. Data shows that donating before surgery only has the potential to make you anemic and at more risk of transfusion. Essentially you are better off keeping your blood to avoid being anemic before surgery.

PAD is also not popular because most people do not end up using the blood and it goes to waste. Self-donated blood cannot go back into the general blood bank so it can't be used by other people. In 1996—during the peak use of PAD—over 60 percent of the donated blood went unused and was discarded. For these reasons, most doctors and current recommendations discourage self-donation prior to surgery as it can make you anemic and often goes unused.

If bleeding is more than expected, a blood transfusion may be needed. Each hospital has its own rules for giving a blood transfusion, but typically involves some clinical signs of anemia and a low hemoglobin. Your body will tell us if you need blood. Your vital signs and your ability to do normal things like get out of the bed or walk down the hall take more effort. You may feel excessively weak, tired, or even dizzy signs similar to when you might feel when you have a heavy period. Low iron means low oxygen levels traveling to your heart, brain, and impaired healing. While you may be nervous or uncomfortable about receiving an unknown donor's blood, sometimes it is necessary to prioritize your health and healing.

Most transfusions take place after surgery. If a transfusion is needed during surgery, both the anesthesiologist and your surgeon will collectively decide that a blood transfusion would be in your best interest. While no one takes the risks of blood transfusions lightly, a transfusion can be necessary in certain situations.

When it comes to blood transfusions, many of us can't help but reflect back to the eighties and nineties when fears of infection were front-page news. Thankfully, times have changed, and modern science has made the blood supply very safe—though no medical procedure is 100 percent risk-free. The primary concern of most people is the risk of infection.

Let's break it down with some perspective:

- The risk of contracting HIV from a blood transfusion is 1 in 2,000,000. To put that into context, you're more likely to be struck by lightning.
- The risk of hepatitis B: about 1 in 300,000—less than the odds of finding a pearl in an oyster.

- For hepatitis C, it's 1 in 1,500,000, and as for West Nile virus, the chance is a very small: 1 in 350,000.

Thanks to advanced technology like nucleic acid testing and strict screening protocols, today's blood donations are safer than ever. So, while the risks aren't zero, they're so rare you should feel confident that the blood supply is one of the safest options available if you ever need a transfusion.

One potential side effect of a blood transfusion is the possibility of an immune response. We take this seriously. The reaction can range from a slight fever, hives, a life-threatening fluid buildup in the lungs (pulmonary edema), and anaphylaxis. Fever is rare at about 1 percent of transfusion and allergic reactions are even more rare (0.1 to 0.3 percent). Although there is limited data to support "pretreating" patients with an antihistamine, like Benadryl, and a fever reducer, like acetaminophen, before transfusions to help minimize the risk of fever or allergy, we often do. This can help minimize the rare chance of experiencing a fever or allergic reaction, which can naturally cause concern during the transfusion process.

Anaphylaxis is a severe, potentially life-threatening allergic reaction that can impact your entire body, causing difficulty breathing, swelling of the face, abdominal pain and even unconsciousness. It is a medical emergency. Thankfully, it is rare, occurring in one in twenty thousand to fifty thousand transfusions.

The take-home message is that if needed, a blood transfusion is relatively safe, especially if your body is showing extreme fatigue and abnormal vital signs. Blood is essential to your brain, heart, and overall healing. If you have religious, cultural, or personal reasons for refusing a blood transfusion, it is crucial to inform your surgeon well in advance of surgery. This allows time to optimize your iron levels and review which blood products, if any, are acceptable to you to use in the case of emergency. Having this discussion ahead of time ensures that your care plan aligns with your preferences and medical needs.

Preparing for Pain Management

If your doctor does not bring up postoperative pain management, you should. Just because you have endured years of pelvic pain, endometriosis, or painful periods, doesn't mean you should expect to suffer after surgery as well.

Regardless of the surgical approach—vaginal, laparoscopic, robotic, or open—there will be some discomfort in the next few days to weeks of your recovery. Typically, open procedures are most uncomfortable, while vaginal, robotic, or laparoscopic surgeries are less so. Your experience with pain will also depend on your age, gender, anxiety, and incision size. Managing pain instead of letting pain manage you is crucial to your recovery. It is important that you feel empowered to have this discussion with your doctor. Pain is real and you are not weak for needing to take medication. As a Black woman, I am admittedly particularly sensitive about discussions of pain management after recovery from major surgery. Research supports that people of color and especially women, are often undertreated or ignored when it comes to complaints of pain. The experience of pain is not only much more complicated and subjective than blood pressure or temperature, but also unfortunately tainted by the bias of sexism and racism inherent to our medical system. This "gender pain gap" impacts not only how our pain is experienced but also how it is treated in medical settings.

In the past and admittedly controversially, pain has been considered a "fifth vital sign." This is to suggest that the same way we monitor your blood pressure, heart rate, and oxygen saturation we should also monitor your pain. Therefore, if you experience pain, it should be treated just like we would treat your blood pressure if it was too high or too low. The overuse of strong and addictive narcotics to treat pain played a significant role in the US narcotic epidemic. As a result physicians have been heavily encouraged to not use narcotics. My stance on treating pain is that it is very important to healing, and while narcotics may play a key role in acute pain management, the prescription and use of them should not be indiscriminate or taken lightly. In my experience, poor control of pain can complicate your recovery. Adequate pain management will not only optimize your recovery but also minimize future complications; for example, when your pain is well controlled you are more willing to move and walk more, which is important to prevent blood clots, allows for deep breathing, and reduces your risk of pneumonia. Controlling your pain is going to make the difference in your recovery so don't underestimate your need to control postoperative pain, especially if you have open abdominal surgery.

Together we must weigh the pros and cons about narcotic use as a part of your pain management plan. This includes an open and honest discussion about the benefits and limitations of narcotic use, including the risk of potential misuse, dependence, and overdose as well as more common side effects like constipation, stomachache, and sedation.

Here are some questions to ask your doctor regarding your post-op pain management:

- What is my plan for postoperative pain medication?
- I have tried (insert medication) before and it made me feel (insert symptom(s). Is there anything else I can try?
- What medications will I be given in the hospital? Will these be the same medications I will take at home, and for how long?
- Do I receive a prescription now or before I leave the hospital?
- Will I need stronger medications, like narcotics and what are your policies for refills if I have severe ongoing pain?

* * *

These are the big issues you need to consider when having a hysterectomy. Now, there are other, more rare issues that can present themselves, of course. The point of informed consent, however, is to talk about the unlikely but more common concerns we have for this surgery. The reality is that your surgery is going to be uncomplicated, but this conversation is an important formality. It helps get the nerves and anxiety out in a calm and organized way.

While all of this may seem overwhelming, remember to take things step-by-step. There are many considerations when deciding to have a hysterectomy and the steps preceding surgery. Deciding what type of hysterectomy, the recovery process, and what to expect will help you feel more prepared. After thoroughly understanding the realistic risks, benefits, and alternatives to surgery you will be better equipped to manage your nerves and ease any anxiety. Once the preoperative steps are complete and your health is optimized, you will arrive on your surgical day feeling informed, empowered, and ready to embrace the rest of your life.

11

❧

Welcome to the OR

Conquering Your Surgical Day Like a Boss

Congratulations! This day has been a long time coming. You've made the empowering decision to take control of your health and undergo a hysterectomy. The days before your surgery are all about preparation and relaxation—both physically and mentally. You will likely feel a mix of emotions as your surgery day gets closer—excitement, anxiety, even relief. That's perfectly normal. Remember all the work you did to get to this point. Remember your reasons for coming to this decision. Know that you are surrounded by a talented team dedicated to your care and well-being.

Let me help take the mystery and unknowns out of the day of your surgery—and the days leading up to it—so that you can feel as comfortable and confident as possible. This chapter is designed to guide you through each step of your hysterectomy experience with clarity. Remember, you're not just having surgery—you're taking control of your health and well-being, and that's a journey worth celebrating.

The Days Leading Up to Surgery

If you are having a vaginal, laparoscopic, or robotic procedure you are likely to be discharged the same day as your surgery, but you should talk with your doctor about this. If you are having an open hysterectomy, you will likely stay one to three nights in the hospital. In any case, you may want to pack a bag with some things to help make your visit more comfortable.

Here are some "do not forget items" for your hospital stay:

- A book or your favorite music or podcast can help keep you occupied while you wait in the preoperative area.
- You may want to have an external battery or extra-long cord so you can keep your phone charged.
- Earplugs, especially if you are staying overnight.
- An eye mask to block out harsh hospital lighting.
- Comfortable, loose-fitting clothing for your hospital stay.
- Essential items like your ID, insurance card, house shoes, and toiletries, including your hair bonnet or pillowcase.

If you are recovering alone, it can help to set some things up ahead of your surgery:

- Make some meals and freeze them ahead of time. Usually warm, nourishing soups and stews full of veggies and protein are the way to go. You can just heat them up over the stove or in the microwave. Stock up on easy breakfasts and snacks, too.
- Do your laundry, clean, and tidy up. You shouldn't be bending over and lifting things while you recover, so plan to get your laundry done and whatever tidying up would help you feel at home in your space before your surgery. Or, conversely, let heavy lifting chores and cleaning wait awhile. Those dust bunnies will still be there in a few weeks when you're feeling better, I promise. Prioritize your recuperation.
- Get your pain medications delivered, and make use of delivery services for other things, too. Or make a quick pharmacy run to

pick up your pain medications, and also options for constipation, earplugs for the hospital, toiletries, and any other knickknacks you may need for comfort.

• Before your surgery, set up a side table or utility cart near a comfy chair, couch, or your bed with things you'll need while you rest: a full water bottle, snacks, a good book, the remote control, your phone charger, dressings for your incisions (if needed), silicone sheets for keloid prevention, lotions to keep your skin moisturized, and your pain medication.

For My Curly Queens: Presurgery Hair Prep Tips

Getting ready for surgery? Don't forget about your beautiful curls! A protective style can be your best friend during your recovery and keep your hair low-maintenance and stress-free. The last thing you want to manage is your hair when you should be healing. Consider cornrows, individual braids, a weave, or a high bun. Remember, you'll be lying on your back during surgery and recovery so your hairstyle should not interfere with your head directly contacting the surgical table or the full range of motion for your neck.

Choose Your Support Person

Feel free to arrive at your appointment alone, but most hospitals require that someone be available to pick you up after your surgery. This person(s) can usually wait with you before surgery and sit at your bedside after you wake up post-surgery.

It is important to choose this person ahead of time. It should be someone you trust and feel comfortable with, especially since it is likely they may hear parts of your medical history and details about the procedure. Your chosen support person can play an essential role as your advocate, helping to communicate with medical staff, family, and friends.

More than that, they'll be a familiar face, a comforting presence, and maybe even a hand to hold as you navigate this part of your journey. Choose wisely—it's a relief to have someone by your side.

Expect a Phone Call from the Hospital the Day Before Your Surgery

The day before the surgery a nurse from the hospital will call you. They may call from a hospital number or blocked line, so consider not sending any calls to voicemail the day before your procedure. Their job is to provide important information you will need for the day of surgery—be sure to take notes.

This will include:

- Instructions on where and when to arrive. Typically plan to arrive two hours before your surgery. There is a registration process that often absorbs this time so please be prompt.
- They will confirm the planned surgery and review the medical history that was provided by your doctor's office. If there are new updates, they will communicate any special needs to your doctor and the operating room staff prior to your arrival.
- They may provide special instructions for you to follow. For example, they will review any medication you are currently taking and remind you to pause medication(s) that may cause bleeding or that your PCP asked you to not take prior to surgery.
- You may be reminded to wash with a special soap or shave if your surgeon prefers that practice.

You may also be asked to start fasting at midnight. Nulla per os (NPO), or fasting, has been standard practice for decades. Why? When there is food in your stomach it can pass into your lungs as you are receiving anesthesia. This is called aspiration and is a serious and preventable anesthesia-related complication.

The American Society of Anesthesiologists (ASA) guidelines have recently relaxed on fasting and drinking prior to surgery and some surgeons and hospitals are adopting these changes. The hospital representative may tell you it is okay to drink clear liquids within the recommended fasting time. This has been a huge shift in practice. We still avoid solid food, but the shorter fasting time and the ability to drink clear liquids is a win-win for you. Each hospital and surgeon have their protocol so please follow the guidelines they provide for you.

Clear liquids include water, sports drinks, coconut water, and tea. Clear liquids are not coffee with cream and milk, a smoothie, or any other drink you cannot see through. Having solid food or non-clear liquid, especially dairy, hours before surgery is a good way to have your procedure canceled or delayed by at least eight hours so be sure to follow these instructions.

Nourish Your Body

Your body is strong. Your body is capable. But for the upcoming journey she is going to need some serious nutrition. Preparing for surgery is not the time to try out new foods or experiment with bold culinary adventures. Instead, stick with meals that are familiar to you—foods that won't surprise you with an unexpected stomach upset. In the days leading up to surgery, focus on light and healthy meals. Protein and vegetables should take center stage on your plate, as your body will rely on these building blocks to repair and heal itself in the weeks ahead.

It's also crucial to address an often overlooked challenge of surgery: constipation. Anesthesia and narcotics commonly used during and after surgery are known to slow down your intestines, potentially leading to uncomfortable bloating and gas. By eating fiber-rich foods, staying hydrated, and preparing ahead of time, you can help your body avoid the unnecessary discomfort of a sluggish system.

Be sure to take your regular medications as scheduled unless your primary care physicians advised you to pause certain medications in the days or weeks prior to surgery. Typically, you will be asked to take your standard medications for hypertension, thyroid disease, or diabetes or modify these according to your doctor's instructions.

Nurture Your Mental State

As you move through the day and days before your surgery, remember that your mindset matters: Everyone manages stress and anxiety differently. Some of us like to be surrounded by friends and family while others like to spend time alone. Whatever works best for you is what you should do. Whether it is a brunch the day before, a massage, yoga class, meditation, or even a long walk, take some time to prioritize your mental health for the journey ahead. Remember that you're making a powerful choice for your health and future well-being. As you drift off to sleep, visualize how much better you'll feel once your symptoms are relieved. You're taking a step that will improve your quality of life, and that's something to celebrate.

Surgery Day

How exciting—we're here! Surgery day has arrived. While every hospital may differ slightly in their approach, the process is fairly standardized and designed with your safety and comfort in mind.

One thing you might notice is some repetition during your check-in and presurgery steps. This is intentional! From verifying your health information to confirming the surgical plan, this repetition is how we dot all the Is and cross all the Ts to ensure everything is accurate and aligned. It's a vital part of creating a safe, smooth, and successful surgical experience.

Take a deep breath—you've got this. Let's walk through the process together.

Arrival and Check-in

As instructed, you and your support person should plan to arrive at the hospital at least two hours early. This gives you time to check in and complete any last-minute registration or insurance paperwork. You will receive a plastic hospital bracelet on your arm with your identifying information, such as your name, date of birth, and your medical record number. The admissions staff will guide you through the process with care and compassion with the understanding that you may be nervous.

Preoperative Area

After check-in, you'll be directed to the preoperative area. These can be large bustling rooms filled with nurses and doctors preparing for surgery. When you enter this space, you will likely see small, partitioned spaces with numbers hanging from the ceiling. Here is where you will wait with your support person as the preoperative nurse starts preparing for your big day. The nurse will hand you a hospital gown and a small sterile cup for a urine sample. Even if you are postmenopausal, some facilities require a pregnancy test. Humor them and provide a small sample.

The nurse will take your vital signs and review of your medical and surgical history. They will review the last time you had anything to eat or drink and perhaps start an IV line that will later be used for fluids and medications. Once your admission to the hospital is completed by the preoperative staff you are likely to have some downtime. During this time, you can lock up your belongings in a locker or a security team will secure them for you. Take this time to read, rest, or meditate. Soon, you will start your interactions with your healthcare team.

The Dream Team

You may not meet all of these folks or know them by name, but you're going to have a whole team working to support you. Let's get acquainted with your medical team and how they will work to keep you safe and comfortable in the OR.

Your Surgeon's Surgical Sidekick: The Gynecological Resident

If you are at a teaching hospital, your surgeon may be working with an ob-gyn resident. While they are still in training, these doctors are learning from the best—your surgeon. If you have concerns about residents, express them, but be reassured they are closely observed by your surgeon. Allowing them in your procedure is not only contributing to the education of future ob-gyns, but also playing a role in advancing medical knowledge. It is challenging to do any surgery alone and their assistance is critical. They will also be your first source of comfort and peace of mind during your hospital stay so please be open to them.

While you are waiting in the perioperative area, the residents are responsible for taking your medical and surgical history. Yes, again. Sorry, I did say it was repetitive. They assist the nurse in making sure all of your preoperative testing and paperwork is completed. The resident may also be the person who consents you for the surgery. This will cover some of the same information you discussed with your doctor in the office so it will not be the first time you hear about the risks, benefits, or alternatives of surgery. Most importantly, during this conversation they can help calm any last-minute nerves by answering questions you may have about the procedure and next steps.

After your surgery, the gynecology resident continues to be an important part of your care team. They'll check on you in the recovery room, monitor your vital signs, and manage any immediate postoperative concerns. They will notify your doctor of how you're recovering immediately postoperative and during your hospital stay. As you recover in the hospital, they'll be a familiar face, checking on your progress, adjusting medications as needed, and coordinating with the rest of your healthcare team to ensure your recovery is on track.

The Orchestrator: The OR Circulating Nurse

Your operating room nurse, otherwise known as your circulating nurse, is a bit of an unsung hero of the operating room. They work hard to keep things flowing and to keep you safe. In the preop area they are the last and final check that everything is in proper order for your surgery. This starts with reviewing your history—yes, I know, again. They will confirm that you have signed the surgical consent and that the surgery on the consent form is in fact the surgery that you have agreed to. They are there to answer any last-minute questions or concerns you have before moving to the operating room. Once in the operating room they help settle you on to the operating table ensuring you are warm and comfortable. The OR nurse will then help position your body to accommodate any knee or back concerns you have expressed.

During the surgery, the circulating nurse helps everyone. They assist the surgeon with instruments and set up equipment so that we can focus on you. They help the anesthesiologist with medications or instruments to keep you safe while under anesthesia. They properly package and label any specimens and make sure they are delivered to pathology for evaluation. During surgery, they spend hours floating between everyone in the room to make sure they have everything they need to enable a seamless procedure.

Your circulating nurse keeps everyone in communication and on the same page about your progress. As you wake up from anesthesia, they will prepare to transfer you to recovery and will give important details about you and your procedure to the nurses that will accept responsibility for your post-op care.

Instrument Maestro: Your Surgical Scrub Technologist

You won't meet your surgical scrub technologist, or scrub tech, until you enter the OR because they are busy preparing the operating room for you. If the resident is our right hand, the surgical scrub tech is our left hand. While you are in the perioperative area, they are in the OR setting up for your surgery. They are responsible for keeping the operating room sterile.

When you enter the OR you will identify them by the hair cap, face mask, and sterile gown they are wearing. Your scrub tech will introduce themselves by their first name and masked smile. After you are asleep, the scrub tech will prepare the surgical site in a sterile fashion and help place drapes to keep your surgical team from touching any other part of your body that is not sterile. They help your surgeon put on their surgical gown and gloves.

Their key role, however, is to pay attention to the surgery and hand the surgeon tools as we ask for them. A good surgical tech can anticipate the surgeons next steps and is always ready with the correct instrument or suture. When they are prepared it helps us minimize your surgical and anesthesia time. Most importantly, their readiness allows your surgeon to focus on what they do best—taking care of you. When done with the surgery, they help us make sure that all the instruments and needles are accounted for. They help clean your surgical site, place any dressings that are required, and get you transferred to the recovery room safely.

The Comfort Commando: Your Anesthesiologist

Before entering the OR your anesthesiologist will introduce themselves and—you guessed it!—ask you questions about your medical history. Their questions will focus on your minor and major past experience(s) with anesthesia. Your answers may influence the type of anesthesia you receive and the medications they do or don't use while you are asleep. They will ask about medications that you are currently taking and medical conditions such as asthma or sleep apnea. This is the time to inquire about any anesthesia-related concerns you might have. They will not only answer your questions, but also explain the process of receiving anesthesia. They will ensure that you feel comfortable and secure before signing the consent form to receive anesthesia.

Your anesthesiologist will then go to the operating room where they will prepare your medication. Once you are in the OR she will place sensors on your chest that monitor your heart rate and rhythm and a blood pressure cuff to monitor your blood pressure throughout the surgery. Heads-up, the first squeeze on the cuff can be uncomfortably tight. Don't worry—it's simply the machine "getting to know you"—rest assured the cuff will not get this tight again. A small monitor or sticker called a pulse oximeter (or pulse ox for short) will also be placed on your finger to measure your oxygen level during the surgery. All these monitors work together to keep tabs on your vital signs while you are sleeping. Once you are safely off to sleep, the anesthesiologist will use this information to monitor your vitals, adjust medications, and collaborate with your surgeon to monitor concerns like blood loss.

When your procedure is completed, the anesthesiologist will slowly remove the sedation. When you are breathing on your own the breathing tube will be removed, and you will wake up safely and comfortably. They will be there to address any immediate postoperative pain, monitor your vitals and any changes in your health while in the recovery phase. After surgery, if you have any discomfort the anesthesiologist will collaborate with your surgeon, nurse, and residents to develop a personalized pain management plan that ensures a smooth and comfortable recovery.

Creative Solutions to Complex Pain Management
When you speak to the anesthesiologist, it's your opportunity to express any concerns about immediate postoperative pain. While no procedure is entirely pain-free, the goal is to effectively and safely control your pain so you can recover smoothly.

Your anesthesiologist and healthcare team are there to help you manage pain in the safest and most attentive way possible. Years of endometriosis and fibroid-related pain may have left you with a complex regimen of pain medications, including the use of narcotics. While this is common, it can make your postoperative pain management a bit more challenging. This isn't just about the medications you've taken—it's also about your unique pain history and how conditions like anxiety, depression, or other psychiatric conditions can amplify the pain perception. These factors are critical for your anesthesiologist to understand, as they can directly influence your recovery experience.

In understanding your exposure to pain medications, your anesthesiologist can help recommend a multispecialty team approach that can effectively address your postoperative pain needs. This may include a team of doctors from pain management, neurology, interventional radiology and even psychiatry to address your pain. Some patients require a truly collaborative approach to address postoperative pain issues.

If you are a complex pain patient, you may consider a preoperative consultation with the anesthesia service prior to your procedure. They can discuss methods of anesthesia and post-op pain relief that are not as often used but possibly effective. The first is patient-controlled analgesia or PCA. This is a range of methods typically associated with an infusion of medication attached to a programmable machine that allows you to administer your own pain relief. The pump can deliver both a steady flow and an extra dose(s) of pain medication as needed. When programmed by the anesthesiologist and working as intended, there is an unlikely risk of overdosing the medication.

A more recent option for longer acting pain relief is called the transversus abdominis plane (TAP) block. A TAP block is a one-time delivery of local long-acting anesthesia delivered into the layers of the muscle. Using an ultrasound, the anesthesiologist injections this medication into the layers of abdominal muscle. Several studies have looked at TAP block in both laparoscopic and open abdominal surgeries. These studies found that patients who receive a TAP block require fewer doses of narcotics in the first twenty-four to forty-eight hours after surgery compared to those who did not have a TAP block.

These are just a few of the anesthesia and pain management options available to you. It's important to remember that you have the right to comprehensive and individualized care when it comes to managing your pain. Start by having an open and honest dialogue with your anesthesiologist and healthcare team. Share your pain history, concerns, and goals for recovery. Together, you can explore the treatments that best suit your needs, whether it's advanced techniques like TAP blocks or patient-controlled analgesia.

Managing complex pain isn't a solo journey—it takes a collaborative team effort involving specialists who are dedicated to your comfort and well-being. With the right plan in place, you can confidently take control of your healing journey and achieve a better quality of life after surgery.

Entering the Operating Room: Showtime in the OR

When it's time for surgery, you'll be escorted by the circulating nurse to the operating room (OR). This is where the magic happens—where you take the final step toward reclaiming your health.

You and your surgeon will likely walk down the hall to the OR together—a moment that feels surreal for many. As we walk toward the OR, you will notice that the temperature drops. No, you are not imagining this. The OR is kept cool, which maintains sterility and keeps equipment in top condition, so it is normal to feel the chill. As the OR door swings open it is easy to get overwhelmed. The room is full of bright lights and you'll see a variety of equipment that might look straight out of a sci-fi movie. You might even hear some music playing softly in the background—an OR tradition to help the team stay focused and relaxed.

But here's the most important thing: every single person in that room is focused on one thing—your safety and well-being. Each team member has a specific role, working together to ensure your procedure goes as smoothly as possible. So, while it might feel like a whirlwind at first, you're in expert hands.

You'll be positioned comfortably on the operating table, where the team will roll out the red carpet of care just for you. First, you'll be wrapped in a warm blanket to keep you cozy.

Next, a resident will place sequential compression devices (SCDs) on your legs—fancy stockings designed to prevent blood clots. You'll feel them gently squeeze your calves as you lay back, like a mini leg massage during your procedure. Your circulating nurse will ensure every detail is just right, carefully cushioning your back and other pressure points to keep you comfortable. Meanwhile, your anesthesiologist will place monitors on your chest, keeping a close eye on your heart, breathing, and vitals.

Then comes the soothing part: we'll ask you to imagine your favorite vacation spot or happiest memory while the anesthesiologist slowly begins administering anesthesia. The sensation of drifting off to sleep will come faster than you expect—and as you do, you can rest assured knowing you've surrounded yourself by a skilled, compassionate team.

This moment isn't just about the procedure—it's the first step in your journey to feeling better and reclaiming your health. You're in capable hands, and we're here to guide you every step of the way.

12

And That's a Wrap

Recovery, One Day at a Time

You wake up, groggy but aware of the soft beeping of the heart monitor beside you. Wrapped under a toasty blanket, welcome to the recovery room, also known as the post-anesthesia care unit (PACU).

The recovery nurse notices you're starting to stir and quietly comes to your bedside. She reassures you with a calm voice, "You're in recovery, sweetheart. Your surgery went well." That simple sentence feels like a hug for your soul.

You'll probably drift off again, your body still under the influence of anesthesia. When you wake up the second time—about an hour later feeling less groggy as the anesthesia continues to wear off.

As your senses sharpen, you might notice a twinge of discomfort in your belly or a slight burn in your throat from the breathing tube, but mostly, you'll feel thirsty. Your nurse will be there with a sip of water, the first you've had in what feels like forever. That cool, refreshing sip is pure bliss.

It's done. Your uterus has left the building, and you are officially in the recovery phase. You may have lots of thoughts and emotions during this time. Most frequently, my patients report a sense of relief. Others feel anxious and wonder, what is next? Well, what's next is simple: healing. There's no need to jump ahead or overthink the road ahead. Take one step, one breath, and one moment at a time. Your body has done the hard work, and now it's time to let it recover—with you giving it the care and patience it deserves.

Your first recovery phase is all about making sure your body is stabilizing after surgery. This includes regular vital signs, warding off nausea (a common post-op symptom), and aggressive pain management. Once you're fully awake, your support person will be allowed to see you, providing you much-needed comfort and reassurance.

Same-Day Discharge After Laparoscopic/Robotic or Vaginal Hysterectomy

What happens next really depends on the type of surgery you have. If you have had a laparoscopic, robotic, or vaginal hysterectomy you may be on the express train home. The resident will come to assess your recovery and communicate with your doctor if you are stable for discharge. This basically means you have met a few important postoperative milestones:

- **Your pain is well controlled:** Your oral pain management is working and your discomfort can effectively be managed at home.
- **You can keep light food down without nausea or vomiting:** Even if your appetite is not fully back, you can safely be discharged to home if you keep down small bits of food and can tolerate liquids.
- **You were able to urinate:** After removal of the catheter, your bladder has to work properly before you can leave, but some centers do not have this as a requirement.
- **You can stand and walk without dizziness:** Mobility is key, but take it slow! Feeling stable is a requirement for discharge.

Once you meet these goals you will likely be fast-tracked home. Remember that everyone will have a different recovery. If anything seems a bit out of order, you may be admitted for the night. Everyone will have a different recovery, so remember this is a marathon not a sprint.

Hospital Stay Recovery: It's a Sleepover . . . Except in the Hospital
If you have an abdominal or open hysterectomy, go ahead and settle in. Over the next few days, your care team—the nurse, resident, and surgeon—will keep an eye on you to make sure you are achieving your post-op goals which make for uncomplicated recovery and planned discharge within one to three days of your surgery. Be kind to your body and communicate with your healthcare team about your recovery. Concentrate on recovery and understand that you can go at your own pace.

Hospital days one to three will focus on meeting the following milestones prior to discharge:

- **Wound care:** Over the next few days, your team is going to make sure there are no bleeding or signs of infection.
- **Eating and drinking:**
  - Begin with clear liquids like water, broth, or electrolyte drinks. Move to solids only when you feel ready. If you have nausea, ask for anti-nausea medication early. Nausea can lead to vomiting, which can be painful on a new and healing abdominal incision.
  - Focus on small manageable bites. You actually may lose weight after surgery, many people do. Your appetite may be a little blunted and this is okay, as long as you can hydrate and take in small amounts of food.
- **Wake up, Ms. Bladder:** After surgery, the Foley catheter will be removed. Once it is out, you will be encouraged to get up and go to the bathroom, first with support from your nurse and then on

your own. This is a sign that your kidneys are functioning and the sensation to your bladder has returned.

- **Passing gas (yes, it is important)**: We are not trying to be vulgar, but let's talk about gas—also known as flatus, which, believe it or not, makes us really happy. After surgery, we will frequently ask if you're passing gas because it is a key sign your gastrointestinal system is waking up. Passing gas signals that the risk of a bowel slow-down (called an ileus, which is when the small intestine slows down after surgery) or complete shutdown (a small bowel obstruction, or SBO) has passed. Passing gas is a reassuring sign everything is moving along as it should. You may not have a bowel movement prior to discharge and that is okay if you are passing gas, eating, and drinking well.

- **Pain management**: Pain management is going to be a big part of your hospital stay. Please do not try to "tough it out." It is important to take your medications on schedule. This means—at the minimum—taking acetaminophen and ibuprofen in four-to-six-hour intervals, along with any other stronger pain medications as needed if your discomfort becomes more intense. Over the first twenty-four hours, you will transition from IV to oral pain meds so be sure to let your care team if your regimen is not working or any adjustments are needed.

- **Walk, walk, rest**: Walking is an incredible jumpstart to your recovery, but you must also rest. It is fine to start small. Your first trip will be to the bathroom, followed by around your room, and then down the hall. Walking will help prevent complications like blood clots and pneumonia. Just as important as walking is rest. Give yourself permission to rest—it is also essential to your healing.

Recovering at Home

The hospital has its purpose, but it is not always the ideal place for healing. Your best recovery will start when you enter your own home, sleep in your own bed, and eat your own food. Your discharge instructions will include all the important instructions on what you need, but here's a more extensive guide of the dos and don'ts that will get you through recovery at home.

- Light activity around the house and even walking outside is highly encouraged. Remember, you are not on bedrest and in fact, movement helps prevent those dangerous complications we've talked about. Think of it as gently waking up your body every day and your effort to not become deconditioned from your procedure.

- If an abdominal binder is comfortable, wear one for added support on your abdomen especially while you are walking. It can provide gentle pressure on your abdomen to help reduce pain with movement.

- Avoid heavy lifting, bending, twisting, or strenuous chores like heavy cooking and cleaning. When a patient asks me how much they can lift I typically say, "Stick to things like your remote control or a fluffy pillow." This is about protecting your incision and abdominal muscles from developing a hernia.

- Even if you are not using stronger pain medications, continue to alternate with over-the-counter medications like acetaminophen and ibuprofen. With time, you will notice a slow improvement in your pain and decreased need for pain medication.

- Do not drive until you have stopped taking narcotics. It is important that you feel strong and alert while driving. Lean on your support system and let friends and family help drive you around. We don't always lean on our support the way we should and you know it. This is a perfect opportunity to let your village support you.

- Keep your incision clean and dry—there is no need to use special creams or lotions on your incision at this time. You can feel comfortable taking a simple shower and gently drying your incision. Watch for signs of infection—warm skin, redness, a foul odor, or drainage and contact your doctor with any concerns. Make sure you follow up with your doctor no later than two weeks to inspect your incision(s) and remove any bandages.

- Listen to your body. Fatigue is normal, but excessive fatigue may be a sign of postoperative anemia. Your natural intuition will tell you that being lightheaded, dizzy, or having chest pain is not normal. You need to report any of these symptoms to your healthcare team immediately.
- Be proactive about your bowel health. Between anesthesia and narcotics you should almost expect some degree of constipation. Plan ahead by adding a stool softener, green leafy vegetables, and lots of water into your routine to help combat painful bloating and constipation.
- Gas pain can make you cry. Consider starting anti-gas medicine soon after surgery and take regular walks. Gentle walks, ginger ale, and chewing gum can also be great for helping let the gas out—these are old wives' tales that definitely has some merit.
- Taking it easy is the basic theme of your recovery phase. For at least 4 to 6 weeks you should really take advantage of this downtime. Let your body heal and remember strenuous activity also includes intercourse—keep everything out of your vagina including douching, tampons, and especially intercourse.

At the end of ten to fourteen days, you should have a follow-up visit scheduled to examine your incision and remove your surgical covering. How you care for your wound after surgery is crucial and reporting signs of infection early are important. Here are the key points to caring for your incision(s) postoperatively, especially if you have melanin-rich skin or are prone to scarring.

- **Keep the incision clean and dry:** This helps prevent infection, which can worsen scarring.

- **Avoid picking at the scabs or rubbing the wound:** Allow the wound to heal naturally. No special creams or lotions are needed for proper healing.

- **Keep the wound covered:** For the first few weeks the incision may be covered with a dressing or a liquid adhesive until the skin closes. Once the skin is closed you can keep it to air without any special dressing unless directed by your surgeon.

- **Consider using silicone sheets:** Silicone-based products are one of the most effective treatments for preventing and minimizing keloid scars. These come in sheets, gels, or creams—I prefer patients use the sheets. You can apply directly over the incision once it's healed. Silicone sheets help prevent raised or thickened scars by creating a moist environment that stimulates collagen, reduces inflammation, and protects from bacteria.

- **Avoid sun exposure:** New scars can become hyperpigmented or darken in the sun. Once your skin is closed you can use topical sunscreen with SPF 30 or higher on your scar and wear protective clothing if you spend much time outside with the incision exposed to the sun.

- **Massage the scar:** Some incisions can respond to massage. After the incision has healed (typically a few weeks after surgery), you can gently massage the scar with moisturizing lotion or cream to disrupt collagen fibers than can cause keloid formation.

- **Pressure therapy:** Some surgeons favor pressure garments to help not only provide abdominal support but also to help flatten the scar and reduce keloid formation.

- **Steroid injections:** If you notice the skin starts to raise, consult your surgeon or dermatologist early to address the potential for keloids. They will often start steroid injections that can help minimize scar formation. The treatments work best if the keloid is early in its formation. If you are known to keloid, ask your surgeon about injecting steroids to prevent keloid formation at the time of surgery.

Pro Tip for Pain Management

Set several alarm reminders on your phone for your medication. It is important in the first few days after a surgery that you do not miss a dose. It's important to keep a steady level of pain relief in your system to help you move around comfortably, which is an essential part of your recovery.

As your body heals and you feel stronger, you'll naturally find yourself needing less medication. Until then, let those reminders take one task off your plate—you've got enough to focus on!

You Were So Brave, Now Recover

You've made it through, and that took incredible courage. Making the decision to have a hysterectomy is no small feat, and now is the time to honor your body by letting her heal. Waking up after surgery marks the start of a new chapter—one of recovery, renewal, and rediscovery.

Whether you're heading straight home or spending a brief stay in the hospital, remember that recovery is a process and an important part of your journey. Be gentle with yourself, follow your doctor's guidance, and take it one step at a time.

Each day will bring you closer to feeling like your fabulous self again. You've got this, and you are so worthy of the care and kindness you show yourself.

13

I Got 99 Problems, but
My Uterus Ain't One

Around six weeks after your surgery (or sooner, if you had a vaginal or laparoscopic procedure) you'll truly start to see the light at the end of the tunnel. This is especially true if you had an abdominal hysterectomy. The discomfort of surgery is gone, and you are starting to get back into the groove of your regular life. Hallelujah!

The post-recovery stage is all about rediscovering your energy and feeling more like your old self again—minus the bleeding and pain, of course. The hardest part is behind you so celebrate your victory. Keep doing what you have been doing including listening to your body and taking recovery at your own pace. You are closer than ever to a future free of uterus-related problems.

Reaching the six-week mark of recovery may feel like a major milestone. At this time, it is normal to think that you are good and done with recovery, but unfortunately for some this might not be the case. Time and time again, I have heard from patients that they wished someone had talked about life after hysterectomy. They felt that while their body was healing beautifully, there were still aspects of post-recovery life and thriving that remained unanswered and they felt uncomfortably uninformed. That's what this chapter is all about. The "now what?" of life after hysterectomy.

The things you may or may not have considered about life after hysterectomy including sex, sexuality, libido, or the feelings that may come up including your new relationship to parenthood, if that interests you. For many of us, there come these intrusive thoughts that creep in from the culture that suggest we are somehow "different," "less feminine," "less desirable" after a hysterectomy. You are not alone in feeling this way, but all these thoughts could not be further from the truth. We will explore these feelings and experiences together.

Embracing Your Feelings

As with all the stages of this process, it's normal to have lots of feelings about your life after hysterectomy. These emotions can vary from person to person. You may have feelings of relief, excitement, and even satisfaction if you have been released from years of pain and heavy bleeding. On the other hand, you may feel loss, sadness, or even significant depression—especially if your uterus was removed for cancer, during pregnancy, or after giving birth.

If you were focused on researching and preparing to make this decision, the buildup and climax of surgery may have left little room for any emotional processing of all of this. Now, in the stillness of recovery and quiet nights after surgery, there may be more time to reflect on your experiences and sit with your feelings. For some this can be overwhelming.

If you had a gender-affirming hysterectomy, you may feel gender euphoria—the feeling of joy and satisfaction when your gender identity finally aligns with how you "see" and experience yourself. You may feel like you're discovering yourself again, or for the first time—this can bring up a lot of conflicting and repressed emotions as you navigate this new experience.

Across all types of hysterectomies, there is not only the journey to recovery, but if you had your ovaries removed, there are also hormonal changes along with the emotional and physical recovery of surgery. This can be a lot to handle. These changes can be profound, and it is not always easy to process them all at once. I clearly remember my own mother trying to navigate recovery with the sudden onset of menopause. The night sweats, hot flashes, and mood changes along with the intensity of recovery was certainly more than she (or us) bargained for. She would alternate between grief, joy, uncertainty, and even relief so quickly it was an emotional roller coaster for everyone in the family. It is okay to release and sit in those feelings, share them, acknowledge them, and ask for support as you navigate this new phase of life.

Your mental health is just as important as your physical health as you live life after a hysterectomy. Emotional ups and downs are normal after surgery. Working through all these feelings can take time. One of the most important and helpful postoperative acts is to give yourself grace. Grace to give yourself permission to take all the time you need both physically and emotionally to recover. Grace to accept that you do not always have to be strong or resilient. Grace to take off the superwoman cape that you have been wearing for decades that has kept you from taking care of yourself while you pour deeply into others—often at your own expense, and to feel whatever you feel.

Talking through your feelings—in therapy, support groups, or even with close friends—is one of the best ways to prioritize your mental health. Creating a space to share and be heard can make a huge difference in how you process your emotions and heal. With each week, you may make it a point to take naps, walk outside, get a massage, practice yoga, or anything else that takes you away from the hustle of your day-to-day. These personal acts of self-care help you recenter yourself and remind you that healing is not just about your physical body. Years of health issues require a reset for your heart, mind, and spirit as well. Rest, ask for support, and take life one gentle and intentional step at a time.

Let's Talk About (Post-Op) Sex, Baby

Regardless of the type of hysterectomy, your doctor will recommend no sex for at least six weeks and while this may seem like a long time, it is actually very standard practice. No sex primarily means no penetration. The primary reason for this is that while the incision on your abdomen may appear to be healed, there is still internal healing taking place and penetration can disrupt this process leading to serious consequences.

If you had a total hysterectomy, penetration can also interrupt the upper part of the vagina or vaginal cuff which was sewn together after the uterus was removed. The thrust of penetration can interrupt internal structures that are still healing, which can lead to internal bleeding, infection, pain, and even the risk of repeat surgery. If you had a subtotal hysterectomy—meaning the cervix is still present—penetration will still be discouraged. Thrusting can still disrupt internal healing. So, while you may (or may not) be eager to resume intimacy, either way please just wait for your doctor's green light. The potential risks are not worth the short-term pleasure.

It's not just sexual penetration that is going to get the red light during this time. Your vagina is on a temporary time out from having anything inserted, as we've discussed. This includes douching—which is not recommended anyway—tampons, and sex toys. While your surgery puts a pause of certain activity, consider it a temporary pause and not a lifetime full stop. Once you are cleared from your doctor, you are free to get right back into the groove of life and relationship.

Reclaiming Pleasure After Hysterectomy

There are plenty of ways to connect sexually during your recovery that don't involve penetration. If you have not had surgery on your external genitals—either a labiaplasty (plastic surgery on the genitals) or perineoplasty (reconstruction of the small area of skin between your lower vagina and rectum known as the perineum)—you are welcome to explore other non-penetrative types of stimulation. Kissing, gentle touch, and simulation of your genital erogenous zones are all fine and orgasm is totally safe. Oral sex is also on the table. If you did have surgery on your external genitals, it is understandable to be cautious when touching these areas. This added precaution likely won't be a difficult request as most people are not interested in touching the skin while it is still healing. As with any activity, go at your own pace and listen to your body.

Once you have received the green light on all activities, you may still not feel ready to take the plunge into penetrative sex. That is entirely reasonable. My patients often have anxiety about pain or tenderness in their abdomen, or as one woman put it, fear of "breaking her vagina." Rest assured that resuming sex is okay. For some, however, you may have to consider exploring ways to help relax yourself as intimacy sex becomes familiar and enjoyable again.

Take it step-by-step. If you are feeling anxious, consider the following:

1. **Start slowly.** There is no need to rush or culminate your first post-surgery sexual experience with penetration. You can work up to this with time. Reconnect in other physical ways and rest assured you will get back to your usual activity soon.
2. **Use lubrication.** If you have never used lubrication before this is a good time to experiment with the many types of lubricants available. If your ovaries have been removed, you may experience a slight decrease in natural lubrication. Even if you have your ovaries, over time a slight decrease in lubrication is normal in everyone. A lack of lubrication can lead to pain which eventually will make you cringe at the thought of being intimate. Invest in a quality water or silicone—which is preferred-based lubricant to reduce discomfort and increase pleasure.
3. **Experiment with different positions.** When you are ready for intimacy but perhaps are a little hesitant, consider positions that do not allow for the deepest penetration. For example, you could try a side lying position with your outer leg in an "L" position, sitting in a chair, or on top of your partner to personally control the depth of penetration.
4. **Stop if there is pain.** While this may seem like a no-brainer, some people are accustomed to pushing through pain during sex and need

to be reminded that sex should not hurt. If you are uncomfortable do not continue. Take your time to relearn your erogenous zones and what gives you pleasure. When you are ready, you can reconsider penetration. If pain or discomfort persists despite time and effort, be sure to check with your physician sooner rather than later.

For everyone, the journey back to sex and intimacy is a personal one. There is no rush. Most commonly, my patients say they are able to return to a healthy sex life and rediscover even more pleasure as they are no longer worried about pain, bleeding, or the thought of pregnancy. Take it step-by-step and take time to rediscover your body on your own terms.

Libido in the Lost and Found: How to Rekindle Your Fire

Sex after a hysterectomy is one thing, but what about your desire and libido? These two issues are a bit more complex, but so very important to your mental and physical well-being. For some people, getting reacquainted with their body has been a lifelong journey. Hysterectomy or not, there is no six-week deadline for that. While research is rich in this area, we continue to still struggle with all the components that influence desire as the need for sex and intimacy change from moment to moment and person to person. Desire and libido are influenced by a myriad of issues that change throughout your lifetime including your relationship status, medication use, health issues and more. Libido can vary with your self-image, relationship satisfaction, communication with your partner, your partner's sexual performance, your libido prior to surgery, and a multitude of other factors. Perhaps your desire will come back with ease and for others it may take some time—both scenarios are normal.

In my professional experience, most patients who have a hysterectomy to address bleeding, fibroids, or endometriosis report an overwhelming improvement in their sex life. For many the journey to reclaiming intimacy may be complex and may take time, but the results are often life changing. For the first time in years they are free of long, painful periods and the constant worry of bleeding or pain interrupting the spontaneity of sex. For them, their hysterectomy allows them to begin separating their negative association of pain and blood with sex. Endometriosis patients are often overjoyed to not have pain with penetration and are eager to try sexual positions that previously provoked pain and anxiety. Not only do they report more satisfaction with sex, there is more or better orgasm. Research supports this experience: Most patients who were sexually active before surgery have the same or better sexual functioning after the surgery.

For cancer patients, the experience may be different. A cancer diagnosis alone is enough to impact one's sexual health. Furthermore, cancer treatments such as radical hysterectomy, radiation, and chemotherapy can cause additional challenges to sexual functioning. Younger cancer patients face the negative impact of these treatments more profoundly with a more significant impact on sexual health. Standard chemotherapy can impact self-image (hair and weight loss), sexual interest (fatigue and vaginal pain), and decrease lubrication. Radiation can narrow, shorten, and dry the vaginal canal which directly causes pain and impacts orgasm. If you are struggling to reignite your libido post-hysterectomy, especially after a cancer diagnosis, know that you are not alone. Your sexual health reboot is going to take a holistic approach including medication, physical therapy, psychotherapy, sex therapy, time and a dedicated effort from you and your partner. It's not easy but it is possible.

The Complex World of the Female Libido

Your libido is not just about what is happening "down there." It is a maze of connections between your body, the pleasure centers of your brain, your satisfaction with your relationship, your desire and need for intimacy, hormonal status, and the real desire to avoid pain. The return of your libido takes time and work. Here are some things to consider:

- **Minimize stress:** I can hear your annoyance through these pages. Are you serious? Easier said than done, I know. The very experience of surgery and life on its own is stressful. Cancer is stressful. Navigating your healthcare and balancing your role as caregiver, community leader, breadwinner and more is stressful. I understand. Stress comes at you from all sides. Your libido, however, is always the first to take a hit. Prioritize your joy and peace. Practice saying "no" to people and activities that do not spark joy and make more space that uplifts and relaxes you.

- **Communicate with your partner:** Your feelings about the change in your body, your healing incisions, and having a hysterectomy can be positively influenced by support from your partner. Keeping lines of communication between you and your partner open often helps with the mental stimulation and emotional intimacy that is important to reignite your libido.

- **Seek professional help:** The benefit and impact of couples and personal sexual therapy cannot be underestimated. Regardless of the reason for a change in your libido counseling is a large part of reestablishing intimacy in a relationship and rediscovering your libido.

- **Consider hormones:** If your ovaries are removed, discuss your options for hormone replacement therapy including testosterone—which may help your libido—with your healthcare team.

- **Lubrication for the win:** Even if you are a candidate for hormonal therapy, do not underestimate the importance of a high-quality lubricant. As mentioned, silicone-based lubricants are ideal, but water-based lubricants are an option as well. Try several options and keep your favorite in your nightstand for easy access.

- **Celebrate erotica:** It is often important to connect with yourself before you can engage with anyone else. The world of erotica, including books, video, and toys, can be an important tool in helping you stimulate the pleasure centers in your brain and body before worrying about anyone else.

- **Self-pleasure is ahhhh-mazing:** Consider exploring personal toys designed for clitoral stimulation and vaginal penetration. Clitoral stimulation uses vibration and/or sucking sensation to increase blood flow to the clitoris making it more likely that you can experience orgasm. Penetrative toys can be inserted into the vagina or rectum and come in various materials, sizes, and shapes. The vagina is muscle and if not used—like any other muscle—will become tighter and narrower especially after some cancer treatments. Regular use of clitoral and penetrative toys paired with lubrication, time, and relaxation techniques will increase blood flow to the vagina and help improve its elasticity.
- **Explore medication for libido:** Speak to your doctor about several medication options for low libido, also known as hypoactive sexual desire disorder (HSDD).
- **Give yourself grace:** Above all, be kind and loving to yourself during this time. Rekindling your libido and relationship takes time but is entirely possible.

Pelvic Floor Rehab: A Strong Pelvic Floor Is Always in Style

Your sexual health extends beyond lubrication and orgasm; sometimes after a hysterectomy your pelvic floor needs some tender loving care too. After a hysterectomy, one of the best things you can do is invest in an evaluation with a pelvic floor therapist. Pelvic floor physical therapy can help strengthen the muscles we take for granted, improve your bladder control, and make intimacy more comfortable.

Your pelvic floor is one of the most underappreciated and overlooked muscle systems of your body. Some women notice that their pelvic floor has improved after hysterectomy, reporting an improvement in their bladder and bowel complaints, and some women even report their sexual health concerns are better as soon as six months after surgery. Others may find their pelvic floor problems got worse, especially those related to the bladder function or vaginal prolapse. This change in pelvic function could be due to a shift in anatomy now that the uterus is gone or perhaps due to a post-surgery change in blood supply or innervation that can lead to a small but present pelvic floor weakness. We more commonly see a weaker pelvic floor in older women, those who are overweight, and those who have had vaginal deliveries—all known risk factors for a compromised pelvic floor.

Fortunately, pelvic floor physical therapists are more accessible than ever, and I highly recommend seeking one out before, but definitely after your surgery. Pelvic floor therapists are trained to help with the treatment of scar tissue, pain relief, improve posture, and even help you improve your breathing. A pelvic floor therapist will provide personal feedback on your pelvic floor and play a valuable role in your post-hysterectomy healing.

* * *

After a few weeks of experimentation, play, and maybe even professional support you should find yourself back where you started in your sexual journey—or in an even better place!

When Pain Persists: Time to See Your Doctor

Understanding the type of pain you are experiencing can help you and your doctor identify the underlying issue.

Superficial Dyspareunia

Superficial dyspareunia is pain with intercourse that occurs with penetration. It may feel like an intense burning or tearing sensation. We can often see superficial dyspareunia after a hysterectomy as the result of a decrease in estrogen if the ovaries are removed or if there is a loss in vaginal moisture. Pain can also occur if any stitching outside the vagina has not healed. Additionally, this pain can happen if surgery or cancer treatments narrow the vaginal opening making penetration uncomfortable.

As a response to this pain, some people may develop a condition known as vaginismus, an involuntary muscle spasm that interferes or prevents any penetration of the vagina. Vaginismus often becomes a reflex response to any attempts at sex or intimate touch, leading to a cycle of tension and discomfort. If vaginismus is present, it cannot be fixed overnight. Treatment of vaginismus requires the coordinated approach, involving a sexual therapist, a pelvic floor specialist as well as the topical estrogen and lubrication to allow the body to unlearn its aversion to pain with sex.

Before vaginismus becomes a concern, report any symptoms of pain or discomfort to your doctor. Your doctor will examine you and if sutures are present or healing is incomplete, you will be advised to hold off on sex until healing is complete. Often six weeks is sufficient, but occasionally more time is needed. If any signs of infection are present, then antibiotics will be prescribed to treat the area.

For issues with dryness, ask your doctor about vaginal estrogen. Vaginal estrogen—which is not the equivalent of hormone replacement therapy—can help improve vaginal dryness, itching, and burning you may be experiencing and is generally safe, even if you have a history of cancer. In addition to vaginal estrogen, you can consider water and silicone lubricants can also help reduce the friction associated with penetration. Lubrication and vaginal estrogen can be helpful after hysterectomy and especially if you are approaching or are in menopause. Lubrication should be used with every interaction even if you are using vaginal estrogen.

Deep Dyspareunia

The second type of pain with sex is known as deep dyspareunia, which can develop differently than superficial dyspareunia. Patients with deep dyspareunia often describe pain or discomfort deeper in the vagina or lower pelvis. They often describe a sensation of something being hit or moving deep inside their body. After a hysterectomy an exam is important to make sure there is no breakdown of the vaginal sutures that can contribute to this sensation.

Although rare, it is important to rule out the possibility of infection. Imaging such as ultrasound or CT scan is typically used to look for infection. If an infection is suspected then antibiotics, possible drainage of the infection, and time will typically resolve your discomfort. Another possible cause of deep dyspareunia is the development of internal scar tissue that may have developed since your surgery. The scar tissue can be provoked when the cervix is removed or as the vaginal cuff heals. Unfortunately, this type of scarring or adhesion is hard to identify on exam or with imaging. Fortunately, typically this type of pain will resolve spontaneously with time. Pelvic floor therapists can help address possible trigger points, adhesions, or other pelvic floor dysfunction associated with deep dyspareunia. In rare cases, a "look and see" diagnostic laparoscopy may be considered if the pain is intense, unrelenting, and does not resolve with any other conservative treatment. This decision, however, is considered a last resort.

The O Show: When Your Finale Feels Far Away

It is important to discuss your orgasmic experience with your surgeon prior to your surgery. Most women (96 percent) achieve orgasm from clitoral stimulation, while a significantly smaller percentage (4 percent) report the ability to orgasm with deep vaginal stimulation. If you typically orgasm with deep vaginal penetration or cervical stimulation it is possible that your sexual experience may change post-hysterectomy. If you have orgasmic dysfunction before your hysterectomy, it may persist or even worsen after surgery.

There is mixed data regarding orgasms after hysterectomy. In general, simple hysterectomies should not impact your orgasm. Radical hysterectomies, however, require extensive dissection around the bladder and pelvis could result in an impact on your orgasm by interrupting the nerves involved in the pathways that allow for your heightened sexual response and orgasm. If your ability to orgasm has become diminished or impacted after a hysterectomy, you should discuss this concern with your doctor as soon as you notice the issues. While only a few women experience these issues, when it happens it can be very unnerving.

If you struggled to have an orgasm prior to your surgery and no hormonal or anatomic issues could be identified, it is imperative to explore psychological or emotional factors that may influence your ability to orgasm. A psychologist, psychiatrist, or sex therapist may be helpful. Medications such as SSRIs (selective serotonin reuptake inhibitors) or other antidepressants can impact orgasm and should be explored with your healthcare team. Sometimes you may consider a change in medication that alleviates this side effect. You and your doctors should also explore medications that may help with orgasm and libido. Hormone replacement therapy—including testosterone—should be considered along with psychotherapy in the form of personal, relationship, and sex counseling to support your journey. If this is your situation, try and view your change in experience as a shift in experience and not a downgrade. Allow yourself time to heal, seek professional health, and practice patience. Most patients return to their normal state over time, but everyone and everybody is unique.

Natural vs. Surgical Menopause

Perimenopause, the several years of time before menopause when estrogen levels start to fluctuate, and menstrual cycles are unpredictable and erratic, and menopause, defined as the day after one year of no menstrual cycles are natural events. Natural menopause is typically a gradual decline in hormone production until you are producing the lowest levels of estrogen of your lifetime. Even when your periods cease, your ovaries continue to produce small amounts of hormones, including testosterone. This testosterone not only impacts libido for years after menopause, but it also converts to estrogen which can help mediate some menopausal symptoms and contribute to bone, brain, and heart health. While natural menopause can be physically challenging, surgical menopause is a different animal entirely.

Surgical menopause causes an abrupt fall in estrogen, progesterone, and testosterone in the body. Almost overnight your body is deprived of these critically important hormones. The sudden loss of these important hormones can be physically, emotionally, and mentally devastating to some women. I still think of the challenges my mother faced navigating a sudden surgical menopause and how the experience is more intense due to the sudden and complete drop in estrogen. Although there are no randomized trials, a large amount of observational data suggests that removal of the ovaries before menopause is associated with a higher rate of death as well as the more rapid progression of eighteen chronic health diseases associated with aging.

Estrogen Replacement Therapy: What You Should Know

If you are a good candidate to receive estrogen, estrogen replacement therapy (ERT) may be the antidote to bothersome menopausal symptoms and mitigate the negative health effects of surgical menopause on your body. Estrogen comes in many forms—oral pills, transdermal patches (absorbed through the skin), or vaginal (creams, pills, and rings). If you are considering or facing removal of the ovaries for health reasons—as a quality-of-life issue—it is critical to discuss the role of estrogen in your post-hysterectomy life with your healthcare team or a menopause specialist. For many people, ERT can help you continue feeling like yourself, as it offers quick relief from the most common symptoms of menopause: vasomotor symptoms, or VMS. VMS, also known as hot flashes or night sweats, are described as a sensation of spontaneously and quickly burning from the inside. During a hot flash—which can last from a few seconds to minutes—your body tries to find a way to cool down, leaving you feeling flushed and sweating. Night sweats, which occur during sleep, are similar to hot flashes that can be so intense that it can leave you drenched.

While ERT is primarily for the use of vasomotor symptoms, if you are young, ERT can help protect your bones from osteoporosis and fractures which can be dangerous and improve heart health by enhancing good cholesterol (HDL) and lowering unfavorable cholesterol (LDL).

This can reduce the risk of cardiovascular disease in women early in menopause. Vaginal estrogen can also help treat vaginal dryness and help support your libido by minimizing painful sexual experiences.

Most leading women's health organizations agree that women under sixty who are within ten years of menopause are often good candidates for ERT, particularly if the ovaries are removed before natural menopause.

You should avoid estrogen therapy if you have:

- a history of stroke
- a history of blood clots, deep vein thrombosis (DVT), or pulmonary embolism (PE)
- heart disease or previous heart attack or stroke
- an unexplained vaginal bleeding
- liver disease
- an estrogen-sensitive cancer (e.g., breast cancer—although this should be individualized)
- a history or high risk of any disease that causes blood clots

As a menopause specialist, I advocate for hormone therapy in people who are appropriate candidates. Like any treatment, ERT is not "one-size-fits-all." It is crucial that you and your healthcare team work together to weigh the benefits and risks to determine what path is right for you.

If estrogen therapy isn't right for you, or if you prefer a nonhormonal approach here are some complementary alternatives:

- **Lifestyle changes:** Regular exercise, a balanced diet rich in calcium and vitamin D, avoiding smoking, and limiting alcohol can go a long way in protecting your bones and heart after menopause. Reducing your alcohol in particular can help reduce vasomotor symptoms.
- **Nonhormonal medications:** There are FDA-approved medications, such as selective serotonin reuptake inhibitors (SSRIs) and

selective estrogen receptor modulators (SERMs), that can help alleviate menopause symptoms without using estrogen.

- **Herbal supplements:** Supplements like black cohosh, soy, or red clover may provide symptom relief, though it's important to discuss these options with your doctor to ensure these supplements are safe for you.
- **Vaginal estrogen:** For vaginal dryness or urinary symptoms, local estrogen treatments (creams, pills, or rings) can offer significant relief with minimal systemic risks.
- **Neurokinin 3 (NK3) receptor antagonists:** A newer class of medications that target the temperature regulating center of the brain by blocking a protein called neurokinin 3, a known trigger of vasomotor symptoms.

Menopause is a natural phase of life, but surgical menopause is not. Please discuss your plan for management of surgical menopause with your healthcare team to find the best path forward for your health and quality of life.

New Paths to Parenthood

A hysterectomy, whether planned or as an emergency, lifesaving procedure doesn't mean that you have to let go of your dreams of becoming a parent. For some, modern science can still help you explore potential paths to parenthood. With that said, I want to keep it real with you—while there are options, the cost can be a significant barrier to achieving your goal. Nevertheless, understanding your options and any potential obstacles will help you make sense of the journey ahead.

Egg Freezing: Time Capsules for Your Future Family

At the time of your cancer diagnosis, or when considering a hysterectomy for endometriosis or fibroids, your medical team should introduce a conversation about your reproductive future. If you are facing the tough decision to remove your uterus for cancer or other reasons and still desire to grow your family, it is essential to consult with a reproductive endocrinologist to learn about your options for egg freezing. This is especially true for women of color who are less likely to undergo fertility sparing treatments prior to treatment for cancer.

Egg freezing is an important option for fertility preservation in young women regardless of the reason for a hysterectomy. It is achieved by giving injections of two reproductive hormones, follicle-stimulating hormone (FSH) and luteinizing hormone (LH), which stimulate the ovaries to produce more eggs than you would in a natural menstrual cycle. When your ovaries are in a hormonal "overdrive" a minor vaginal procedure is performed to collect each maturing egg before it ovulates. These eggs are then evaluated under a microscope and mature eggs are quickly frozen and stored in liquid nitrogen until they are ready for future use.

If you are considering becoming a biological parent in the future but do not have a partner or sperm donor, egg freezing could be a good option to preserve your fertility, and it tends to not be as large an investment as traditional in vitro fertilization (IVF). A drawback, however, is that there is no guarantee the frozen eggs will go on to create viable embryos and then a full-term pregnancy. For this reason and based on age and other health factors, your doctors may recommend at least a thirty egg retrieval to increase your chances of a successful pregnancy. Generally, the older you are, the more eggs you need to store to help maximize the chances of a live pregnancy. We can also break it down by age. Check out these stats:

- **Women under 35:** freezing 15 mature eggs offers a cumulative 80 percent chance of at least one live birth.
- **Women 35 to 37:** freezing 25 mature eggs offers a cumulative 80 percent chance of at least one live birth.
- **Women 38 to 40:** freezing 30 to 45 mature eggs offers a cumulative 80 percent chance of at least one live birth.

- **Women 40 to 42:** freezing 20 to 30 mature eggs offers a cumulative 50 percent chance of at least one live birth.

In general, the older you are, the more eggs you'll need to bank to maximize your chances of achieving a live pregnancy.

Chillin' with a Purpose: Freezing Embryos, Preserving Possibilities

Like egg freezing, embryo freezing involves hormone injections and monitoring. The big difference is that after the egg retrieval, the eggs are then fertilized with your partner's or donor's sperm. The embryos can then immediately be frozen and kept in storage until you are ready to make reproductive moves.

Embryos have a higher success rate for live birth when they are thawed and transferred than eggs that are stored by themselves. If you have a partner and you both are ready to take a more concrete step toward future parenting, freezing embryos might be the way to go. The cost is slightly higher than that of egg freezing alone because there are extra steps, so you will need to plan accordingly. If you are having a hysterectomy due to cancer concerns, there are often funds that can help support the process.

The Ultimate Team Effort: Surrogacy and the Art of Shared Parenthood

If carrying a child is no longer an option for you, a gestational carrier or surrogacy are two other options you may want to consider. While often used interchangeably, a gestational carrier and surrogate are not the same.

A gestational carrier is someone who carries your pregnancy but is not biologically related to the child. Egg and sperm from the intended parents, or egg or sperm from a donor are used to create an embryo using in vitro fertilization. This embryo is then transferred to the gestational carrier's uterus. Gestational carriers can be found through friends, family, or agencies that specialize in the legal aspects of this process for where you live.

A surrogate on the other hand is biologically related to the child as she uses her own egg during the pregnancy. After delivery, she surrenders her parental rights to the intended parents. Similar to gestational carriers, surrogates can be found through agencies, fertility clinics, surrogacy attorneys, and networking through friends and family. You need to understand the surrogacy laws in your area to understand what your options are.

Finding Family Through Adoption

Adoption is also an option, but you should know that deciding to adopt is a major decision. The adoptee community is very vocal about the complexities of adoption and it is important to learn from them what is needed to establish a healthy adoption for both parties. There are many existing resources to help you learn about the complexities, challenges, and benefits of adoption.

Adoption can take place in several ways, so research is critical to learn which options are available to you. Adoptions can take place domestically, internationally, or through the foster care system. As you can imagine this process can be lengthy as it involves a thorough review of you, your partner, and readiness for adoption. It also is influenced by the age of the child (baby, toddler, teen) you would like to adopt. Once you are approved for adoption the waiting period begins. Eventually, if all goes well, you will match with a birth family or child and the process proceeds from there depending on the adoption route you have chosen.

* * *

The loss of your uterus can be life changing. If you envision becoming a parent, it may feel like the door to this dream has been forever closed. It may be an opportunity to explore a realm of other options and possibilities. Parenthood comes in many packages and there are many ways to explore building your family and define family on your own terms.

You Are So Much More Than Your Uterus

Despite what we are conditioned to believe, the uterus is not the seat of your femininity, sexuality, personal identity, or even power. Your wit, style, humor, and intelligence are your calling card on this earth—not your uterus. You are the same vibrant person you, your family, and friends have always known sans uterus. It is time to redefine womanhood, starting with you.

There is no one-size-fits-all definition of womanhood or personhood—there never has been. Embracing your body in its new form is part of your post-hysterectomy process. You deserve to live freely, experience pleasure, and focus on your mental health.

If you are exploring ways to grow your family like adoption or surrogacy, remember that your path to parenthood is uniquely yours. These experiences are just another stop of your life's journey. If you are exploring your libido and sexuality post-surgery, consider it an opportunity to reconnect with your body and new dimensions of pleasure. You should know that your post-hysterectomy life is full of new possibilities and adventure.

My final word to you—and hear me carefully, because I know each situation is unique—having a uterus is optional, you continuing to be whole, powerful, and uniquely you is mandatory.

Conclusion

A Love Letter from Dr. Kameelah

My dear friend,

You picked up this book because the universe has taken you on a journey that you never expected. Life has handed you a burden that you have had to carry for far too long. I know how heavy that weight has been. What you have endured with your body and what you still might be facing is not only real—it is a lot. You may feel like your body has betrayed you, like the universe hasn't been listening to your cries for relief. I understand the desire deep inside you just to be okay—to just be healthy, to live your life without pain or fear.

You've probably already had to make some incredibly hard decisions, and there are others you're still facing. But let me tell you something: I see you and recognize your bravery, your resilience, and determination to fight for yourself. I honor your strength even when you don't feel strong. I am not asking you to be a superwoman—that trope is dangerous and unrealistic—but I am asking you to stand in your power because you are not broken.

This journey isn't easy, but "hard" doesn't mean you can't win. You are capable, worthy, and deserving of peace in your body and joy in your life. This decision—this moment—is an act of self-love, a step toward reclaiming your health and happiness. So, as you move forward, know this: You're not alone. Please stop suffering in pain or silence. You deserve to live a full life.

I'm here cheering for you, and so is every woman who has walked this path before you. Sis, you've got this. You're stronger than you realize, and you're on your way to the life you deserve. You are my hero.

With love, admiration, and belief in your strength,
Dr. Kameelah

Acknowledgments

This book would not have been possible without the support, guidance, and encouragement of so many incredible people.

To my wonderful patients: Thank you for trusting me with your care and sharing your journeys with me. Your resilience and courage have been my greatest inspiration. Each story you've shared has shaped me and this book. You all have motivated me to create this resource that empowers others facing similar challenges.

I am able to do great things because I stand on the shoulders of my loving friends and family. To my family: Your unwavering love and support have been my foundation. To my grandparents who set the foundation for everything that I am. I love and miss you. To my mother, Cynthia Kennedy, who taught me the power of perseverance and resilience. To my husband, Charles, who will always be my rock and greatest supporter. To my children, Riley, Emory, and Marc, who remind me daily why it's so important to fight for a better future. To the Phillips family who raised me, I love you all so much. To my mentors and colleagues: Thank you for your guidance and for fostering an environment where women's health is a priority. Your expertise and passion for patient care have been instrumental in shaping my perspective and practice.

To my editor, Nana K. Twumasi: Thank you for your vision for this book and for me as the one to spearhead its message, and for all your helpful guidance—and patience—along the way.

To my literary agents Ericka Phillips and Stephanie Tade: Thank you for your advocacy of me and this project through all its ups and downs, and for holding my hand as a first-time author.

To my collaborator, Colleen Martell: Your insight, patience, and dedication turned this vision into reality. Thank you for believing in this project and helping me present it in a way that is both accessible and impactful.

To my friends who are really family: thank you for accepting me as I am. Thank you for being my sounding board, motivation, and cheerleader. You make me a better person.

To the women of color who came before us and gave their bodies to advance women's health: Your courage will continue to inspire generations.

Finally, to anyone who reads this book: Thank you for letting me be a part of your journey. I hope this book empowers and informs you, reminding you that you are never alone in your choices or your healing.

With gratitude and hope,
KPC

Bibliography

AAGL Advancing Minimally Invasive Gynecology Worldwide. "AAGL Position Statement: Route of Hysterectomy to Treat Benign Uterine Disease." *Journal of Minimally Invasive Gynecology* 18, no. 1 (2011).

Aarts, J. W., et al. "Surgical Approach to Hysterectomy for Benign Gynaecological Disease." *Cochrane Database of Systematic Reviews* 8 (2015): CD003677. https://doi.org doi: 10.1002/14651858.CD003677.pub5.

Aerts, Leen, et al. "Sexual Life After Hysterectomy: Still a Neglected Topic?" *Sexual Medicine Reviews* 8, no. 2 (2020):181182. https://doi.org/10.1016/j.sxmr.2020.03.001.

Ahangari, Alebtekin. "Prevalence of Chronic Pelvic Pain among women: An Updated Review." *Pain Physician* 2;17, no. 2;3 (2014). https://doi.org/10.36076/ppj.2014/17/e141.

Al-Hendy, A., and M. Badr. "Can Vitamin D Reduce the Risk of Uterine Fibroids?" *Womens Health* (London) 10, no. 4 (2014): 353–8. https://doi.org/10.2217/whe.14.24.

Al-Mulhim, Abdulrahman Saleh, et al. "Obesity Disease and Surgery." *International Journal of Chronic Diseases* 2014 (2014): 1–9. https://doi.org/10.1155/2014/652341.

Aliabadi, A. R., et al. "Contraceptive Strategies for Reducing the Risk of Reproductive Cancers." *Obstetrical & Gynecological Survey* 79, no. 10 (2024): 576–77. https://doi.org/10.1097/ogx.0000000000001335.

Alonso, Anais, et al. "Medical Management of Endometriosis." *Current Opinion in Obstetrics and Gynecology* 36, no. 5 (2024):353361. https://doi.org/10.1097/GCO.0000000000000983.

American College of Obstetricians and Gynecologists. "ACOG Practice Bulletin. No. 73: Use of Hormonal Contraception in Women with Coexisting Medical Conditions." *Obstetrics & Gynecology* 107, no. 6 (2006):1453–72. https://doi.org/10.1097/00006250-200606000-00055.

American College of Obestericians and Gynecologists. " ACOG Practice Bulletin No. 114: Management of Endometriosis." *Obstetrics & Gynecology* 116, no. 1 (2010): 223–236. https://doi.org/10.1097/AOG .0b013e3181e8b073.

Aso, Takeshi. "Equol Improves Menopausal Symptoms in Japanese Women." *Journal of Nutrition* 140, no. 7 (2010). https://doi.org/10.3945/jn.109 .118307.

Azadi, A., et al. "Vaginal Hysterectomy Compared with Laparoscopic Hysterectomy in Benign Gynecologic Conditions: A Systematic Review and Meta-analysis." *Obstetrics and Gynecology* 142, no. 6 (2023). https://doi .org/10.1097.

Bailey, Percival. "Hysteria: The History of a Disease." *Archives of General Psychiatry* 14, no. 3 (1966): 332. https://doi.org/10.1001/archpsyc.1966 .01730090108024.

Baird, D. D., et al. "Vitamin D and the Risk of Uterine Fibroids." *Epidemiology* 24, no. 3 (2013): 447–453.

Bansi-Matharu, L., et al. "Rates of Subsequent Surgery Following Endometrial Ablation Among English Women with Menorrhagia: Population-based Cohort Study." *BJOG* 120, no. 12 (2013): 1500–7. https://doi.org/10.1111 /1471-0528.12319.

Barjon, Kyle, and Lyree Mikhail. "Uterine Leiomyomata." StatPearls.com. August 7, 2023. https://www.ncbi.nlm.nih.gov/books/NBK546680/.

Barra, F., et al. "Current Understanding on Pharmacokinetics, Clinical Efficacy and Safety of Progestins for Treating Pain Associated to Endometriosis." *Expert Opinion on Drug Metabolism & Toxicology* 14, no. 4 (2018): 399–415.

Basrai, Zahir. "Tranexamic Acid Treatment for Heavy Menstrual Bleeding." *Journal of Emergency Medicine* 40, no. 4 (2011): 479. https://doi.org/10.1016 /j.jemermed.2011.01.006.

Bedaiwy, M. A., et al. "Medical Management of Endometriosis in Patients with Chronic Pelvic Pain." *Seminars in Reproductive Medicine* 35, no. 1 (2017): 38–53. https://doi.org/10.1055/s-0036-1597308.

Bender, Herman E. "Some Select Vulva Rock Petroglyphs and Forms in North America." *Anthropomorphic Images in Rock Art Paintings and Rock Carvings*, February 27, 2020, 200–214. https://doi.org/10.2307/j.ctv1228gc6.18.

Berntorp, E., et al. "No Increased Risk of Venous Thrombosis in Women Taking Tranexamic Acid." *Thrombosis Haemostasis* 86, no. 2 (2001): 714–5.

Billett, H. H. "Hemoglobin and Hematocrit." In *Clinical Methods: The History, Physical, and Laboratory Examinations*, edited by H. K. Walker, et al. Boston: Butterworths, 1990.

Blair, H. A. "Relugolix/Estradiol/Norethisterone Acetate: A Review in Endometriosis-Associated Pain." *Drugs* 84, no. 4 (2024): 449–457. https://doi.org/10.1007/s40265-024-02018-3.

Bläuer, M., et al. "Vitamin D Inhibits Myometrial and Leiomyoma Cell Proliferation in Vitro." *Fertility and Sterility* 91, no. 5 (2009):1919-25. https://doi.org/10.1016/j.fertnstert.2008.02.136.

Bofill, Rodriguez M., et al. "Interventions for Heavy Menstrual Bleeding." *Cochrane Database of Systematic Reviews* 5, no. 5 (2022): CD013180.

Bruijn, A. M., et al. "Uterine Artery Embolization vs Hysterectomy in the Treatment of Symptomatic Uterine Fibroids: 10-Year Outcomes from the Randomized EMMY Trial." *American Journal of Obstetrics and Gynecology* 215, no. 6 (2016): 745. https://doi.org/0.1016/j.ajog.2016.06.051.

Buck, E., et al. "Menstrual Suppression." StatPearls. com. Updated June 7, 2024. https://www.ncbi.nlm.nih.gov/books/NBK592411/.

Bulkeley, Kelly. "Why Sleep Deprivation Is Torture." *Psychology Today*, December 15, 2014. https://www.psychologytoday.com/us/blog/dreaming -in-the-digital-age/201412/why-sleep-deprivation-is-torture#:~:text=A %20recently%20released%20report%20by,Why%20is%20this?.

Burton, Graham J., and Abigail L. Fowden. "The Placenta: A Multifaceted, Transient Organ." *Philosophical Transactions of the Royal Society B:*

Biological Sciences 370, no. 1663 (2015). https://doi.org/10.1098/rstb.2014 .0066.

Buttram, Veasy C. "Conservative Surgery for Endometriosis in the Infertile Female: A Study of 206 Patients with Implications for Both Medical and Surgical Therapy." *Fertility and Sterility* 31, no. 2 (1979): 117–23. https://doi .org/10.1016/s0015-0282(16)43809-4.

"Cancer Stat Facts: Cervical Cancer." National Cancer Institute. https://seer .cancer.gov/statfacts/html/cervix.html.

Canlorbe, Geoffroy, et al. "Spontaneous Hymeneal Endometriosis: A Rare Cause of Dyspareunia." *BMJ Case Reports*, March 26, 2014. https://doi.org /10.1136/bcr-2013-202299.

Casper, R. F. "Progestin-Only Pills May Be a Better First-line Treatment for Endometriosis Than Combined Estrogen-Progestin Contraceptive Pills." *Fertility and Sterility* 107, no. 3 (2017): 533–536. https://doi.org/10.1016 /j.fertnstert.2017.01.003.

"Cervical Cancer Causes, Risk Factors, and Prevention." National Cancer Institute. Updated August 2, 2024. https://www.cancer.gov/types/cervical /causes-risk-prevention#:~:text=People%20who%20smoke%20or %20breathe,a%20higher%20risk%20of%20cancer.

Chakraborty, Natalie, et al. "Is Total Laparoscopic Hysterectomy with Longer Operative Time Associated with a Decreased Benefit Compared with Total Abdominal Hysterectomy?" *American Journal of Obstetrics and Gynecology* 228, no. 2 (2023). https://doi.org/10.1016/j.ajog.2022.09.042.

Chauncey, J. M., and J. S. Wieters. "Tranexamic Acid." StatPearls.com. Updated July 24, 2023.

Chen, L., et al. "The Multi-functional Roles of Menstrual Blood-derived Stem Cells in Regenerative Medicine." *Stem Cell Research & Therapy* 10, no. 1 (2019).

Chiaffarino, F., et al. "Diet And Uterine Myomas." *Obstetrics & Gynecology* 94, no. 3 (1999): 395–8. https://doi.org/10.1016/s0029-7844(99)00305-1.

Cianci S., et al. "Exploring Surgical Strategies for Uterine Fibroid Treatment: A Comprehensive Review of Literature on Open and Minimally Invasive

Approaches." *Medicina* (Kaunas, Lithuania) 60, no. 1 (2023): 64. https://doi.org/10.3390/medicina60010064.

Cichowski, S. B., et al. "Sexual Abuse History and Pelvic Floor Disorders in Women." *Southern Medical Journal* 106, no. 12 (2013): 675–8. https://doi.org/10.1097/SMJ.0000000000000029.

Coleman, E., et al. "Standards of Care for the Health of Transgender and Gender Diverse People, Version 8." *International Journal of Transgender Health* 23, no. sup1 (2022). https://doi.org/10.1080/26895269.2022.2100644.

Collaborative Group on Epidemiological Studies of Ovarian Cancer. "Ovarian Cancer and Oral Contraceptives: Collaborative Reanalysis of Data from 45 Epidemiological Studies Including 23,257 Women with Ovarian Cancer and 87,303 Controls." *Lancet.* 371, no. 9609 (2008): 303–14.

Colman, Drew E. et al. "Patient and Surgery Characteristics of Inpatient Hysterectomies among Transgender Individuals." *LGBT Health* 10, no. 7 (2023): 544–51. https://doi.org/10.1089/lgbt.2022.0388.

Committee on Gynecologic Practice. "Committee Opinion No 701: Choosing the Route of Hysterectomy for Benign Disease." *Obstetrics & Gynecology* 129, no. 6 (2017): e155–e159. https://doi.org/10.1097/AOG.0000000000002112.

Cooper, D. B., and G. W. Menefee. "Dilation and Curettage." StatPearls.com. Updated May 7, 2023. https://www.ncbi.nlm.nih.gov/books/NBK568791/.

Cooper Owens, D. B. *Medical Bondage: Race, Gender, and the Origins of American Gynecology.* University of Georgia Press, 2017.

Cox, Emily. "Embryology, Ovarian Follicle Development." StatPearls.com, August 14, 2023. https://www.ncbi.nlm.nih.gov/books/NBK532300/.

Critchley, H. O. D., et al. "Physiology of the Endometrium and Regulation of Menstruation." *Physiology Review* 100, no. 3 (2020): 1149–1179.

Czuczwar, P., et al. "The Influence of Uterine Artery Embolisation on Ovarian Reserve, Fertility, and Pregnancy Outcomes—a Review of Literature." *Menopause Review* 15, no. 4 (2016): 205–209. https://doi.org/10.5114/pm.2016.65665.

Dedden, S. J., et al. "Hysterectomy and Sexual Function: A Systematic Review and Meta-analysis." *Journal of Sexual Medicine* 20, no. 4 (2023):447–466. https://doi.org/10.1093/jsxmed/qdac051.

DeLancey, J. O., et al. "The Appearance of Levator Ani Muscle Abnormalities in Magnetic Resonance Images After Vaginal Delivery." *Obstetrics and Gynecology* 101, no. 1 (2003): 46–53. https://doi.org/10.1016/s0029-7844(02)02465-1.

Dewi, F. N., et al. "Endogenous and Exogenous Equol Are Antiestrogenic in Reproductive Tissues of Apolipoprotein E-null Mice." *Journal of Nutrition* 142, no.10 (2012):1829–35 https://doi.org/10.3945/jn.112.161711.

Dietz, H. P., and B. Clarke. "Prevalence of Rectocele in Young Nulliparous Women." *Australian and New Zealand Journal of Obstetrics and Gynaecology* 45, no. 5 (2005): 391–4.

Dominoni, M., et al. "Which Is the Best Surgical Approach for Female-to-Male Sexual Reassignment? A Systematic Review of Hysterectomy and Salpingo-Oophorectomy Options from the Gynecological Perspective." *Medicina* (Kaunas, Lithuania) 60, no. 7 (2024): 1095. https://doi.org/10 3390/medicina60071095. PMID: 39064524; PMCID: PMC11278962.

Donnez, J., and P. Jadoul. "What Are the Implications of Myomas on Fertility?" *Human Reproduction* 17, no. 6 (2002): 1424–30. https://doi.org /10.1093/humrep/17.6.1424.

Doyle, Joseph O., et al. "Successful Elective and Medically Indicated Oocyte Vitrification and Warming for Autologous In Vitro Fertilization, with Predicted Birth Probabilities for Fertility Preservation According to Number of Cryopreserved Oocytes and Age at Retrieval." *Fertility and Sterility*, 105, no. 2: 459–466.e2.

Drogell, Kristin, et al. "Race and Sex Are Associated with Variations in Pain Management in Patients Presenting to the Emergency Department with Undifferentiated Abdominal Pain." *Journal of Emergency Medicine* 63, no. 5 (2022): 629–35. https://doi.org/10.1016/j.jemermed.2022.09.001.

Dye, Christian K., et al. "Psychosocial Stress and MicroRNA Expression Profiles in Myometrial Tissue of Women Undergoing Surgical Treatment for Uterine Fibroids." *Reproductive Sciences* 31, no. 6 (2024): 1651–61. https://doi.org/10.1007/s43032-024-01482-2.

Edwards, M., and A. S. Can. "Progestins." StatPearls.com. Updated January 10, 2024. https://www.ncbi.nlm.nih.gov/books/NBK563211/.

Epelboin, S., and J. Labrosse. "Cultural Perspectives on the Placenta." *Journal of Clinical Images and Medical Case Reports* 4, no. 4 (2024): 1713.

Faramarzi, H., et al. "The Potential of Menstrual Blood-Derived Stem Cells in Differentiation to Epidermal Lineage: A Preliminary Report." *World Journal of Plastic Surgery* 5, no. 1 (2016): 26–31.

Farland, L. V., and A. W. Horne. "Disparity in Endometriosis Diagnoses between Racial/Ethnic Groups." *BJOG* 126, no. 9 (2019): 1115–16. https://doi.org/10.1111/1471-0528.15805.

Fennessy, F. M., et al. "Uterine Leiomyomas: MR Imaging-guided Focused Ultrasound Surgery—Results of Different Treatment Protocols." *Radiology* 243, no. 3 (2007): 885–93. https://doi.org/10.1148/radiol.2433060267.

Florence, Ashley M. "Leiomyoma." StatPearls.com, July 17, 2023. https://www.ncbi.nlm.nih.gov/books/NBK538273/.

Forsgren, Catharina, et al. "Effects of Hysterectomy on Pelvic Floor Function and Sexual Function—a Prospective Cohort Study." *Acta Obstetricia et Gynecologica Scandinavica* 101, no. 10 (2022): 1048–56. https://doi.org/10.1111/aogs.14437.

Gan, T. J. "Poorly Controlled Postoperative Pain: Prevalence, Consequences, and Prevention." *Journal of Pain Research*, no. 10. (2017): 2287–2298. https://doi.org/10.2147/JPR.S144066.

García-Gómez, Elizabeth, et al. "Regulation of Inflammation Pathways and Inflammasome by Sex Steroid Hormones in Endometriosis." *Frontiers in Endocrinology* 10 (2020). https://doi.org/10.3389/fendo.2019.00935.

García-Miguel, F. J., et al. "Preoperative Assessment." *The Lancet* 362, no. 9397: 1749–1757.

Gasner, Adi. "Physiology, Uterus." StatPearls.com, July 30, 2023. https://www.ncbi.nlm.nih.gov/books/NBK557575/.

Geraci, L., et al. "Magnetic Resonance Imaging-Guided Focused Ultrasound Surgery for the Treatment of Symptomatic Uterine Fibroids." *Case Reports in Radiology*, May 3, 2017. https://doi.org/10.1155/2017/2520989.

Gezer, A., and E. Oral. "Progestin Therapy in Endometriosis." *Womens Health* (London) 11, no. 5 (2015): 643–52. https://doi.org/10.2217/whe.15.42.

Giri, A., et al. "Obesity and Pelvic Organ Prolapse: A Systematic Review and Meta-analysis of Observational Studies." *American Journal of Obstetrics and Gynecology* 217, no. 1 (2017): 11–26.e3.

Goldman, R. H., et al. "Predicting the Likelihood of Live Birth for Elective Oocyte Cryopreservation: A Counseling Tool for Physicians and Patients." *Human Reproduction* 32, no. 4 (2017): 853–859. https://doi.org/10.1093/humrep/dex008. PMID: 28166330.

Giromini, C., and D. I. Givens. "Benefits and Risks Associated with Meat Consumption during Key Life Processes and in Relation to the Risk of Chronic Diseases." *Foods* 11, no. 14 (2022): 2063. https://doi.org/10.3390/foods11142063.

Giuliani, Emma, et al. "Epidemiology and Management of Uterine Fibroids." *International Journal of Gynecology & Obstetrics* 149, no. 1 (2020): 3–9. https://doi.org/10.1002/ijgo.13102.

Gleeson, M., et al. "The Anti-inflammatory Effects of Exercise: Mechanisms and Implications for the Prevention and Treatment of Disease." *Nature Reviews Immunology* 11, 607–615 (2011). https://doi.org/10.1038/nri3041.

Graziottin, Alessandra. "Maintaining Vulvar, Vaginal and Perineal Health: Clinical Considerations." *Women's Health* 20 (2024). https://doi.org/10.1177/17455057231223716.

Grimes, W. R., and M. Stratton M. "Pelvic Floor Dysfunction." StatPearls.com. Updated June 26, 2023. https://www.ncbi.nlm.nih.gov/books/NBK559246/.

Guinness World Records. "Strongest Muscle." https://www.guinnessworldrecords.com/world-records/67575-strongest-muscle.

Guo, S. W. "Recurrence of Endometriosis and Its Control." *Human Reproduction Update* 15, no. 4 (2009): 441–61. https://doi.org/10.1093 /humupd/dmp007.

Gupta, C. C., et al. "Sleep Hygiene Strategies for Individuals with Chronic Pain: A Scoping Review." *BMJ Open* 13, no. 2 (2023): e060401. https://doi .org/10.1136/bmjopen-2021-060401.

Harada, T., et al. "Low-Dose Oral Contraceptive Pill for Dysmenorrhea Associated with Endometriosis: A Placebo-Controlled, Double-Blind, Randomized Trial." *Fertility and Sterility* 90, no. 5 (2008): 1583–8. https:// doi.org/10.1016/j.fertnstert.2007.08.051.

Harris, Susan S. "Vitamin D and African Americans," *Journal of Nutrition* 136, no. 4 (2006). https://doi.org/10.1093/jn/136.4.1126.

He, D., et al. "Global Burden of Pelvic Inflammatory Disease and Ectopic Pregnancy from 1990 to 2019." *BMC Public Health* 23, no. 1 (2023): 1894. https://doi.org/10.1186/s12889-023-16663-y.

Hendrix, S. L., et al. "Pelvic Organ Prolapse in the Women's Health Initiative: Gravity and Gravidity." *American Journal of Obstetrics and Gynecology* 186, no. 6 (2002): 1160–6.

"The Historical Significance of Doulas and Midwives." National Museum of African American History and Culture. https://nmaahc.si.edu/explore /stories/historical-significance-doulas-and-midwives.

Hoffman, Kelly M., et al. "Racial Bias in Pain Assessment and Treatment Recommendations, and False Beliefs about Biological Differences between Blacks and Whites." *Proceedings of the National Academy of Sciences* 113, no. 16 (2016): 4296–4301. https://doi.org/10.1073/pnas.1516047113.

Holdsworth-Carson, S. J., et al. "Predicting Disease Recurrence in Patients with Endometriosis: An Observational Study." *BMC Medicine* 22, no. 1 (2024):320. https://doi.org/10.1186/s12916-024-03508-7.

Iolascon A., et al. "Recommendations for Diagnosis, Treatment, and Prevention of Iron Deficiency and Iron Deficiency Anemia." *Hemasphere.*8, no. 7 (2024): e108. https://doi.org/10.1002/hem3.108.

Jackson, L. W., et al, "The Association Between Heavy Metals, Endometriosis and Uterine Myomas Among Premenopausal Women: National Health and Nutrition Examination Survey 1999–2002," *Human Reproduction* 23, no. 3 (2008): 679–87. https://doi.org/10.1093/humrep/dem394.

Jacobs, V. R., et al. "Body Piercing Affecting Laparoscopy: Perioperative Precautions." Journal Am Assoc Gynecol Laparosc. 2004 Nov;11(4):537-41. https://doi.org/10.1016/s1074-3804(05)60089-8.

Janssen, Matthew K., and Steven J. Ralston. "Maternal Morbidity Associated with Multiple Repeat Cesarean Deliveries." *50 Studies Every Obstetrician-Gynecologist Should Know*, January 2021, 103–7. https://doi.org/10.1093/med/9780190947088.003.0019.

Jeldu, M., et al. "Pregnancy Rate after Myomectomy and Associated Factors among Reproductive Age Women Who Had Myomectomy at Saint Paul's Hospital Millennium Medical College, Addis Ababa: Retrospective Cross-Sectional Study." *International Journal of Reproductive Medicine*, November 28, 2021. https://doi.org/10.1155/2021/6680112.

Joshi, Niraj R., et al. "Progesterone Resistance in Endometriosis Is Modulated by the Altered Expression of microRNA-29C and FKBP4." *Journal of Clinical Endocrinology & Metabolism*, October 25, 2016. https://doi.org/10.1210/jc.2016-2076.

Juganavar, Anup, and Ketav Joshi. "Chronic Pelvic Pain: A Comprehensive Review." *Cureus*, October 26, 2022. https://doi.org/10.7759/cureus.30691.

Kahn, Ryan M., et al. "Salpingectomy for the Primary Prevention of Ovarian Cancer." *JAMA Surgery* 158, no. 11 (2023): 1204. https://doi.org/10.1001/jamasurg.2023.4164.

Kamal, D.A.-O., et al. "Beneficial Effects of Green Tea Catechins on Female Reproductive Disorders: A Review." *Molecules* 26 (2021): 2675. https://doi.org/10.3390/molecules26092675.

Kao, Audiey. "History of Oral Contraception," *AMA Journal of Ethics*, June 2000. https://journalofethics.ama-assn.org/article/history-oral-contraception/2000-06#:~:text=The%20Food%20and%20Drug%20Administration,as%20it%20is%20popularly%20known.

Kazemi, F., et al. "Effect of Hysterectomy Due to Benign Diseases on Female Sexual Function: A Systematic Review and Meta-analysis." *Journal of Minimally Invasive Gynecology* 29, no. 4 (2022): 476–488. https://doi.org /10.1016/j.jmig.2021.10.012.

Kenny, M. C., and Wurtele, S. K. "Toward Prevention of Childhood Sexual Abuse: Preschoolers' Knowledge of Genital Body Parts." In *Proceedings of the Seventh Annual College of Education Research Conference: Urban and International Education* edited by M. S. Plakhotnik and S. M. Nielsen, Miami: Florida International University, 2008.

Kim, H. S., et al. "Uterine Rupture in Pregnancies Following Myomectomy: A Multicenter Case Series." *Obstetrics & Gynecology Science* 59, no. 6 (2016): 454–462. https://doi.org/10.5468/ogs.2016.59.6.454.

Koltsova, A. S., et al. "A View on Uterine Leiomyoma Genesis through the Prism of Genetic, Epigenetic and Cellular Heterogeneity." *International Journal of Molecular Science* 24, no. 6 (2023): 5752. https://doi.org/10.3390 /ijms24065752.

Kongnyuy, E. J., and C. S. Wiysonge. "Interventions to Reduce Haemorrhage During Myomectomy for Fibroids." *Cochrane Database of Systematic Reviews*, 11 (2011): CD005355. https://doi.org/10.1002/14651858 .CD005355.pub4.

Kopatsaris, S., et al. "Management of Endometrial Cancer: A Comparative Review of Guidelines." *Cancers* 16, no. 21 (2024): 3582. https://doi.org/10 .3390/cancers16213582.

Kröncke, T. "An Update on Uterine Artery Embolization for Uterine Leiomyomata and Adenomyosis of the Uterus." *British Journal of Radiology* 96, no. 1143 (2023). https://doi.org/10.1259/bjr.20220121.

Küçük, T., and K. Ertan. "Continuous Oral or Intramuscular Medroxyprogesterone Acetate Versus the Levonorgestrel Releasing Intrauterine System in the Treatment of Perimenopausal Menorrhagia: A Randomized, Prospective, Controlled Clinical Trial in Female Smokers." *Clinical and Experimental Obstetrics & Gynecology* 35, no. 1 (2008): 5760.

Kulkarni, A., et al. "Innovations in the Management of Vaginal Cancer." *Current Oncology* 29, no. 5 (2022): 3082–3092. https://doi.org/10.3390 /curroncol29050250.

Kumar, V., et al. "Endometrial Ablation for Heavy Menstrual Bleeding." *Womens Health* 12, no. 1 (2016): 45–52. https://doi.org/10.2217/whe.15.86.

Lacroix, A. E., et al. "Physiology, Menarche." StatPearls.com. Updated March 11, 2023. https://www.ncbi.nlm.nih.gov/books/NBK470216/.

Lähteenmäki, P., et al. "Open Randomised Study of Use of Levonorgestrel Releasing Intrauterine System as Alternative to Hysterectomy." *BMJ* 316, no. 7138 (1998): 1122–6. https://doi.org/10.1136/bmj.316.7138.1122.

Langton, C. R., et al. "Soy-Based Infant Formula Feeding and Uterine Fibroid Development in a Prospective Ultrasound Study of Black/African-American Women." *Environmental Health Perspectives* 131, no. 1 (2023): 17006. https://doi.org/10.1289/EHP11089.

Langton, Christine R., et al. "Family History and Uterine Fibroid Development in Black and African American Women." *JAMA Network Open* 7, no. 4 (2024). https://doi.org/10.1001/jamanetworkopen.2024.4185.

Lanzola, E. L., and K. Ketvertis. "Intrauterine Device." StatPearls.com. Updated June 26, 2023. https://www.ncbi.nlm.nih.gov/books /NBK557403/.

LaVeist, Thomas A., et al. "400 Years of Inequality since Jamestown of 1619." *American Journal of Public Health* 109, no. 1 (2019): 83–84. https://doi.org /10.2105/ajph.2018.304824.

Lee, Jangwoo, et al. "Associations of Exposure to Phthalates and Environmental Phenols with Gynecological Disorders." *Reproductive Toxicology* 95 (2020): 19–28. https://doi.org/10.1016/j.reprotox.2020.04 .076.

Lei, J., et al. "HPV Vaccination and the Risk of Invasive Cervical Cancer." *New England Journal of Medicine* 383, no. 14 (2020): 1340–1348. https:// doi.org/10.1056/NEJMoa1917338.

Leminen, Hurskainen Ritva. "Tranexamic Acid for the Treatment of Heavy Menstrual Bleeding: Efficacy and Safety." *International Journal of Women's Health*, August 17, 2012: 413. https://doi.org/10.2147/ijwh.s13840.

Leserman, J. "Sexual Abuse History: Prevalence, Health Effects, Mediators, and Psychological Treatment." *Psychosomatic Medicine* 67 (2005): 906–15.

Lethaby, A., et al. "Preoperative Medical Therapy Before Surgery for Uterine Fibroids." *Cochrane Database of Systematic Reviews* 11, no. 11 (2017): CD000547. https://doi.org/10.1002/14651858.CD000547.pub2.

Lukes, A. S., et al. "Tranexamic Acid Treatment for Heavy Menstrual Bleeding: A Randomized Controlled Trial." *Obstetrics and Gynecology* 116, no. 4 (2010): 865–875. https://doi.org/10.1097/AOG.0b013e3181f20177.

Lukies, M., and W. Clements. "Current Strategies for Prevention of Infection After Uterine Artery Embolisation." *CardioVascular and Interventional Radiology* 45, no. 7 (2022): 911–17. https://doi.org/10.1007/s00270-022 -03158-3.

Madva, Elizabeth N., et al. "What's All the Hysteria About? A Modern Perspective on Functional Neurological Disorders." *Biological Psychiatry*, January 15, 2019. https://pmc.ncbi.nlm.nih.gov/articles/PMC6444349/.

Marjoribanks, J., et al. "Nonsteroidal Anti-inflammatory Drugs for Dysmenorrhoea." *Cochrane Database of Systematic Reviews* 20, no. 1 (2010): CD001751. https://doi.org/10.1002/14651858.CD001751.pub2.

Maybin, J. A., and H. O. Critchley. "Menstrual Physiology: Implications for Endometrial Pathology and Beyond." *Human Reproduction Update* 21, no. 6 (2015): 748–61.

Mechsner, S. "Endometriosis, an Ongoing Pain-Step-by-Step Treatment." *Journal of Clinical Medicine* 11, no. 2 (2022): 467. https://doi.org/10.3390 /jcm11020467.

Medikare, V., et al. "The Genetic Bases of Uterine Fibroids; a Review." *Journal of Reproductive Infertility* 12, no. 3. (2011):181–91.

Meigs, J.V. "Endometriosis—Its Significance." *Annals of Surgery* 114, no. 5 (1941): 866–74. https://doi.org/10.1097/00000658-194111000-00007.

Michels, K. A., et al. "Modification of the Associations Between Duration of Oral Contraceptive Use and Ovarian, Endometrial, Breast, and Colorectal Cancers." *JAMA Oncology* 4, no. 4 (2018): 516–521. https://doi.org/10.1001/jamaoncol.2017.4942.

Micić, J., et al. "Currently Available Treatment Modalities for Uterine Fibroids." *Medicina* (Kaunas, Lithuania) 60, no. 6 (2024): 868. https://doi.org/10.3390/medicina60060868.

Mijatovic, V., and P. Vercellini. "Towards Comprehensive Management of Symptomatic Endometriosis: Beyond the Dichotomy of Medical Versus Surgical Treatment." *Human Reproduction* 39, no. 3 (2024): 464–477. https://doi.org/10.1093/humrep/dead262.

Minalt, N., et al. "Endometrial Ablation." StatPearls.com. Updated December 19, 2022. https://www.ncbi.nlm.nih.gov/books/NBK459245/.

Mintz, Laurie B., and Kelsi E. Quicksall. *Becoming Cliterate: Why Orgasm Equality Matters —and How to Get It.* New York, NY: HarperOne, 2018.

Moalli, P. A., et al. "Risk Factors Associated with Pelvic Floor Disorders in Women Undergoing Surgical Repair." *Obstetrics and Gynecology* 101, no. 5, pt. 1 (2003): 869–74.

Morrison, Sheena M., and Elizabeth Fee. "Nothing to Work with but Cleanliness: The Training of African American Traditional Midwives in the South." *American Journal of Public Health* 100, no. 2 (2010): 238–39. https://doi.org/10.2105/ajph.2009.182873.

Mukhopadhaya, Neelanjana, et al. "Uterine Fibroids: Impact on Fertility and Pregnancy Loss." *Obstetrics, Gynaecology & Reproductive Medicine* 17, no. 11 (November 2007): 311–17. https://doi.org/10.1016/j.ogrm.2007.08.005.

Nagata, C., et al. "Association of Intakes of Fat, Dietary Fibre, Soya Isoflavones and Alcohol with Uterine Fibroids in Japanese Women." *British Journal of Nutrition* 101, no. 10 (2009): 1427–31. https://doi.org/doi:10.1017/s0007114508083566.

Nelson, G., et al. "Guidelines for Perioperative Care in Gynecologic/Oncology: Enhanced Recovery After Surgery (ERAS) Society Recommendations—2019 Update." *International Journal of Gynecological Cancer* 29 (2019): 651.

Ngernprom, P., et al. "Risk Factors for Recurrent Endometriosis After Conservative Surgery in a Quaternary Care Center in Southern Thailand." *PLOS ONE* 18, no. 8 (2023). https://doi.org/10.1371/journal.pone .0289832.

Odejinmi, F., et al. "Caesarean Section in Women Following an Abdominal Myomectomy: A Choice or a Need?" *Facts, Views & Vision in ObGyn* 12, no. 1 (2020): 57–60.

Olsen, A. L., et al. "Epidemiology of Surgically Managed Pelvic Organ Prolapse and Urinary Incontinence." *Obstetrics and Gynecology* 89, no. 4 (1997): 501–6.

"Operating Room Staff Roles and Responsibilities (in the US)." Incision.com, April 28, 2022. https://www.incision.care/blog/operating-room -department#:~:text=Everyone%20of%20the%20surgical%20team,other %20during%20the%20patient's%20surgery.

Opoku, Albert A., et al. "Challenges of Morbid Obesity in Gynecological Practice." *Best Practice & Research Clinical Obstetrics & Gynaecology*, 90 (2023): 102379. https://doi.org/10.1016/j.bpobgyn.2023.102379.

Orellana, Minerva, et al. "'In Our Community, We Normalize Pain': Discussions around Menstruation and Uterine Fibroids with Black Women and Latinas." *BMC Women's Health* 24, no. 1 (2024). https://doi.org/10 .1186/s12905-024-03008-z.

Orta, O. R., et al. "Dairy and Related Nutrient Intake and Risk of Uterine Leiomyoma: A Prospective Cohort Study." *Human Reproduction* 35, no. 2 (2020): 453–63. https://doi.org/10.1093/humrep/dez278.

Paffoni, A., et al. "Vitamin D Status in Women with Uterine Leiomyomas." *Journal of Clinical Endocrinology & Metabolism.* 98, no. 8 (2013): E1374–E1378.

Pascual, Zoey N. "Physiology, Pregnancy." StatPearls.com, May 16, 2023. https://www.ncbi.nlm.nih.gov/books/NBK559304/.

Patel, D. A., et al. "Childbirth and Pelvic Floor Dysfunction: An Epidemiologic Approach to the Assessment of Prevention Opportunities at Delivery." *American Journal of Obstetrics and Gynecology* 95 (2006).

Patisaul, H. B. "Endocrine Disruption by Dietary Phyto-oestrogens: Impact on Dimorphic Sexual Systems and Behaviours." *Proceedings of the Nutrition Society* 76, no. 2 (2017): 130–144. https://doi.org/ 10.1017/ S0029665116000677.

Pham, TV, et al. "Addressing Chronic Pain Disparities Between Black and White People: A Narrative Review of Socio-ecological Determinants." *Pain Management* 13, no. 8 (2023): 473–496. https://doi.org/10.2217/pmt-2023 -0032.

Pillarisetty, Leela Sharath. "Vaginal Hysterectomy." StatPearls.com, April 24, 2023. https://www.ncbi.nlm.nih.gov/books/NBK554482/.

Pisco, João M., et al. "Pregnancy after Uterine Fibroid Embolization." *Fertility and Sterility* 95, no. 3 (March 2011). https://doi.org/10.1016/j.fertnstert .2010.08.032.

Plosker, G. L., and R. N. Brogden. "Leuprorelin." *Drugs* 48 (1994): 930–967. https://doi.org/10.2165/00003495-199448060-00008.

Lethaby, A., et al. "Preoperative Medical Therapy Before Surgery for Uterine Fibroids." *Cochrane Database of Systematic Reviews*, November 15, 2017.

Puri, N., and A. Talwar. "The Efficacy of Silicone Gel for the Treatment of Hypertrophic Scars and Keloids." *Journal of Cutaneous Aesthetic Surgery* 2, no. 2 (2009): 104–6. https://doi.org/10.4103/0974-2077.58527.

Ramaiyer, Malini, et al. "Menstruation in the USA." *Current Epidemiology Reports* 10, no. 4 (2023): 186–95. https://doi.org/10.1007/s40471-023 -00333-z.

Rawlinson, A., et al. "A Systematic Review of Enhanced Recovery Protocols in Colorectal Surgery." *Annals of the Royal College of Surgeons of England* 93, no. 8 (2011): 583–8. https://doi.org/10.1308/147870811X605219.

Roshdy, E., et al. "Treatment of Symptomatic Uterine Fibroids with Green Tea Extract: A Pilot Randomized Controlled Clinical Study." *International Journal of Women's Health* 7 (2013): 477–486. https://doi.org/10.2147 /IJWH.S41021.

Rosner, Julie. "Physiology, Female Reproduction." StatPearls.com, March 20, 2024. https://www.ncbi.nlm.nih.gov/books/NBK537132/.

Sathe, A., et al. "Medroxyprogesterone." StatPearls.com. Updated February 29, 2024. https://www.ncbi.nlm.nih.gov/books/NBK559192/.

Schilter, Léa V., et al. "Gender-Based Differential Management of Acute Low Back Pain in the Emergency Department: A Survey Based on a Clinical Vignette." *Women's Health* 20 (2024). https://doi.org/10.1177 /17455057231222405.

Shen, Y., et al. "Vegetarian Diet and Reduced Uterine Fibroids Risk: A Case-Control Study in Nanjing, China." *Journal of Obstetrics and Gynaecology Research* 42 (2016): 87–94. https://doi.org/10.1111/jog.12834.

Shim, J. Y., et al. "Use of the Drospirenone-Only Contraceptive Pill in Adolescents with Endometriosis." *Journal of Pediatric and Adolescent Gynecology* 37 (2024): 402–406.

Siegel, R. L., et al. "Cancer Statistics, 2024." *CA: A Cancer Journal for Clinicians* 74, no. 1 (2024): 12–49. https://doi.org/10.3322/caac.21820.

Sirovich, B. E., and H. G. Welch. "The Frequency of Pap Smear Screening in the United States." *Journal of General Internal Medicine* 19, no. 3 (2004): 243–50. https://doi.org/10.1111/j.1525-1497.2004.21107.x.

"Soy Sauce Market Size, Share & Industry Analysis." Fortune Business Insights. Updated January 6, 2025. https://www.fortunebusinessinsights .com/soy-sauce-market-102857.

Spies, J. B., et al. "Uterine Artery Embolization for Leiomyomata." *Obstetrics and Gynecology* 98, no. 1 (2001): 29–34. https://doi.org/10.1016/s0029 -7844(01)01382-5.

Spies, J. B. "Current Evidence on Uterine Embolization for Fibroids." *Seminars in Interventional Radiology* 30, no. 4 (2013): 340–6. https://doi.org/10.1055 /s-0033-1359727.

Spong, C. Y., et al. "Timing of Indicated Late-preterm and Early-term Birth." *Obstetrics and Gynecology* 118, no. 2 pt.1 (2011): 323–333. https://doi.org /10.1097/AOG.0b013e3182255999.

Stewart, E. A., et al. "Clinical Outcomes of Focused Ultrasound Surgery for the Treatment of Uterine Fibroids." *Fertility and Sterility* 85, no. 1 (2006): 22–9.

Stumpf, M. A. M., and M. C. Mancini. "Challenges in the Care and Treatment of Patients with Extreme Obesity." *Archives of Endocrinology and Metabolism* 68 (2024): e230335. https://doi.org/10.20945/2359-4292-2023-0335.

Stoiber, Tasha. "What Are Parabens, and Why Don't They Belong in Cosmetics?" Environmental Working Group. April 9, 2019. https://www.ewg.org/what-are-parabens.

Sundström, A., et al. "The Risk of Venous Thromboembolism Associated with the Use of Tranexamic Acid and Other Drugs Used to Treat Menorrhagia: A Case-control Study Using the General Practice Research Database." *BJOG* 116, no. 1 (2009): 91–7. https://doi.org/10.1111/j.1471-0528.2008.01926.x.

Swift, S., et al. "Pelvic Organ Support Study (POSST): the distribution, clinical definition, and epidemiologic condition of pelvic organ support defects." *American Journal of Obstetrics and Gynecology* 192, no. 3 (2005): 795–806.

Takala, Hajra, et al. "Alcohol Consumption and Risk of Uterine Fibroids." *Current Molecular Medicine* 20, no. 4 (2020): 247–58. https://doi.org/10.2174/1566524019666191014170912.

Thakar R. "Is the Uterus a Sexual Organ? Sexual Function Following Hysterectomy." *Sexual Medicine Reviews* 3, no. 4 (2015). https://doi.org/10.1002/smrj.59.

Till, S. R., et al. "Sexual Function After Hysterectomy According to Surgical Indication: A Prospective Cohort Study." *Sex Health* 19, no. 1 (2022): 46–54. https://doi.org/10.1071/SH21153.

Timmons, Greg. "How Slavery Became the Economic Engine of the South." History.com. Updated March 6, 2024. https://www.history.com/news/slavery-profitable-southern-economy.

Tinelli, A., et al. "Uterine Fibroids and Diet." *International Journal of Environmental Research and Public Health* 18, no. 3 (2021): 1066. https://doi.org/10.3390/ijerph18031066.

Tjeertes, E. K., et al. "Obesity—a Risk Factor for Postoperative Complications in General Surgery?" *BMC Anesthesiology* 15 (2015): 112.

Tollefsbol, Trygve. "Translational Epigenetics Series." *Epigenetics and Reproductive Health* 21, (2021): ii. https://doi.org/10.1016/b978-0-12 -819753-0.09001-2.

Trimble, C. L., et al. "Concurrent Endometrial Carcinoma in Women with a Biopsy Diagnosis of Atypical Endometrial Hyperplasia: A Gynecologic Oncology Group Study." *Cancer* 106, no. 4 (2006): 812–9. https://doi.org /10.1002/cncr.21650.

Turner, K. A., et al. "Disparities in Female Oncofertility Care in the United States: More Questions Than Answers." *Life* (Basel). 13, no. 7 (2023): 1547. https://doi.org/10.3390/life13071547.

van de Wiel, Lucy. *Freezing Fertility: Oocyte Cryopreservation and the Gender Politics of Aging.* New York University Press: 2020.

van der Kooij, S. M., et al. "Uterine Artery Embolization Versus Surgery in the Treatment of Symptomatic Fibroids: A Systematic Review and Metaanalysis." *American Journal of Obstetrics and Gynecology* 205, no. 4 (2011): 317–18. https://doi.org/10.1016/j.ajog.2011.03.016.

van Happs, A. P., et al. "The effect of dietary interventions on pain and quality of life in women diagnosed with endometriosis: a prospective study with control group." *Human Reproduction* 38, no. 12 (2023): 2433–2446. https://doi.org/10.1093/humrep/dead214.

Vandermorris, Ashley, and Daniel L. Metzger. "An Affirming Approach to Caring for Transgender and Gender-Diverse Youth." *Paediatrics & Child Health* 28, no. 7 (2023): 437–48. https://doi.org/10.1093/pch/pxad045.

Vercellini, Paolo, et al. "Estrogen-Progestins and Progestins for the Management of Endometriosis." *Fertility and Sterility* 106, no. 7 (2016). https://doi.org/10.1016/j.fertnstert.2016.10.022.

"Vitamin D." National Institutes of Health. Updated July 26, 2024. https:// ods.od.nih.gov/factsheets/VitaminD-HealthProfessional/.

Waldron, M. G., et al. "Uterine Artery Embolisation of Fibroids and the Phenomenon of Post-Embolisation Syndrome: A Systematic Review." *Diagnostics* (Basel) 12, no. 12 (2022): 2916. https://doi.org/10.3390 /diagnostics12122916.

Walker, W. J., and J. P. Pelage. "Uterine Artery Embolisation for Symptomatic Fibroids: Clinical Results in 400 Women with Imaging Follow Up." *BJOG* 109, no. 11 (2002): 1262–72. https://doi.org/10.1046/j.1471-0528.2002 .01449.x.

Wall, L. Lewis. "The Medical Ethics of Dr. J. Marion Sims: A Fresh Look at the Historical Record." *Journal of Medical Ethics* 32, no. 6 (006): 346–50. https://doi.org/10.1136/jme.2005.012559.

Wall, L. Lewis. "J. Marion Sims and the Vesicovaginal Fistula: Historical Understanding, Medical Ethics, and Modern Political Sensibilities." *Female Pelvic Medicine & Reconstructive Surgery* 24, no. 2 (2018): 66–75. https://doi.org/10.1097/spv.0000000000000546.

Wassenaar, Shannon. "Anatomically Correct Body Part Names: Why It's Important." *Nurtured First*, February 23, 2024. https://nurturedfirst.com /baby/name-body-parts/#:~:text=Using%20anatomically%20correct %20terms%20for,taboo%20around%20those%20body%20parts.

Watrowski, R., et al. "Complications in Laparoscopic and Robotic-Assisted Surgery: Definitions, Classifications, Incidence and Risk Factors—An Up-to-date Review." *Wideochirurigia I Inne Techniki Maloinwazyjne* (Poland) 16, no. 3 (2021): 501–525. https://doi.org/10.5114/wiitm.2021 .108800.

Weisse, C. S., et al. "Do Gender and Race Affect Decisions About Pain Management?" *Journal of General Internal Medicine* 16, no. 4 (2001): 211–7. https://doi.org/10.1046/j.1525-1497.2001.016004211.x.

White, Randall, et al. "Context and Dating of Aurignacian Vulvar Representations from Abri Castanet, France." *Proceedings of the National Academy of Sciences* 109, no. 22 (2012): 8450–55. https://doi.org/10.1073 /pnas.1119663109.

Wise, L. A., et al. "Intake of Fruit, Vegetables, and Carotenoids in Relation to Risk of Uterine Leiomyomata." *American Journal of Clinical Nutrition* 94, no. 6. (2011): 1620–31.

Woodard, Terri L., and Michael P. Diamond. "Physiologic Measures of Sexual Function in Women: A Review." *Fertility and Sterility* 92, no. 1 (July 2009): 19–34. https://doi.org/10.1016/j.fertnstert.2008.04.041.

Yang, F., and Y. Chen. "Urinary Phytoestrogens and the Risk of Uterine Leiomyomata in US Women." *BMC Women's Health* 23, no. 1 (2023): 261. https://doi.org/10.1186/s12905-023-02381-5.

Yang, Q., et al. "Comprehensive Review of Uterine Fibroids: Developmental Origin, Pathogenesis, and Treatment." *Endocrinology Review* 43, no. 4 (2022): 678–719. https://doi.org/10.1210/endrev/bnab039.

Yilma, Hunde Gonfa, et al. "Genistein: Dual Role in Women's Health." *Nutrients* 13, no. 9 (2021): 3048. https://doi.org/10.3390/nu13093048.

Yilma, Hunde Gonfa, et al. "Anti-inflammatory Activity of Phytochemicals from Medicinal Plants and Their Nanoparticles: A Review," *Current Research in Biotechnology* 6 (2023). https://doi.org/10.1016/j.crbiot.2023 .100152.

Yunker, Amanda, et al. "Systematic Review of Therapies for Noncyclic Chronic Pelvic Pain in Women." *Obstetrical & Gynecological Survey* 67, no. 7 (July 2012): 417–25. https://doi.org/10.1097/ogx.0b013e31825cecb3.

Zhang, Y., et al. "Combined Exposure to Multiple Endocrine Disruptors and Uterine Leiomyomata and Endometriosis in US Women." *Frontiers in Endocrinology* 12 (2021): 726876. https://doi.org/10.3389/fendo.2021 .726876.

Zorbas, K. A., et al. "Continuous Versus Cyclic Oral Contraceptives for the Treatment of Endometriosis: A Systematic Review." *Archives of Gynecology and Obstetrics* 292, no. 1 (2015): 37–43.

Index

About the Author

DR. KAMEELAH PHILLIPS is a board-certified ob-gyn with extensive experience in women's health and patient advocacy. Her unique approach combines education, emotional intelligence, cultural humility, and authenticity, making healthcare less intimidating, relatable, and easier to understand for her patients.

Dr. Phillips's passion for women's health stems from her own life experiences. Raised by women in a working-class, multigenerational family, she witnessed firsthand the challenges of medical bias, limited medical education, and inadequate access to quality care. These early lessons taught her the resilient power of matriarchy and fueled her lifelong commitment to empowering women and their families with nonjudgmental, evidence-based care tailored to their individual needs.

Determined to uplift her community, Dr. Phillips pursued her calling in medicine and advocacy. She earned a degree in human biology with an emphasis in women's health and human sexuality from Stanford University and went on to graduate from the University of Southern California Keck School of Medicine, where she received community service and humanitarian awards for her dedication to elevating women globally. Her commitment to advocacy took her on medical missions to Cuba, Ghana, and Tanzania, and she brought lifesaving skills to Haiti during the devastating 2010 earthquake.

During her residency at New York University, she earned surgical honors, laying the foundation for her future work in improving women's health outcomes.

Dr. Phillips's lifelong mission to educate, empower, and inspire women across the diaspora culminated in the opening of her private practice in New York City in 2020 at the height of the COVID-19 pandemic. Delivering care during such a transformative time highlighted the profound health inequities faced by women, further driving her focus on maternal mortality, fibroid management, and menopause care.

With a global perspective and a deep understanding of the systemic barriers to care, Dr. Phillips is a champion for improving access, education, and transparency in medicine. Her work continues to honor the legacy of women's resilience while forging a future of equitable healthcare for all.